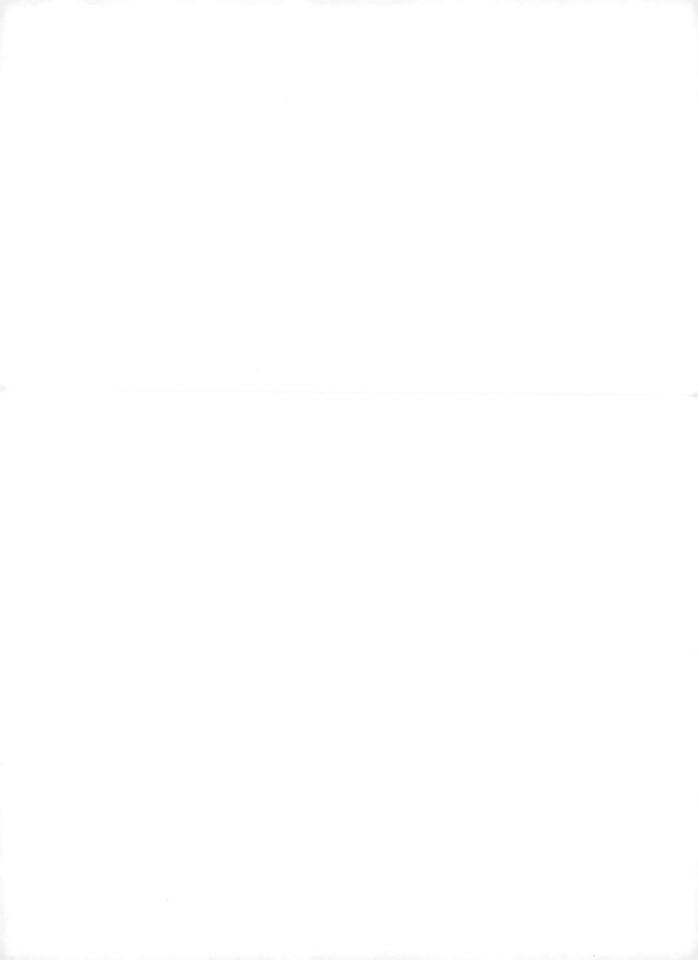

Atlas of
WOMEN'S DERMATOLOGY

From Infancy to Maturity

Atlas of
WOMEN'S DERMATOLOGY
From Infancy to Maturity

Lawrence Charles Parish, MD
Clinical Professor of Dermatology and Cutaneous Biology; and
Director of the Jefferson Center for International Dermatology
Jefferson Medical College of Thomas Jefferson University, Philadelphia; and
Visiting Professor of Dermatology,
Tulane University School of Medicine, New Orleans, USA

Sarah Brenner, MD
Head, Department of Dermatology, Tel Aviv Sourasky Medical Center,
Ichilov Hospital; and Clinical Associate Professor of Dermatology,
Sackler School of Medicine, Tel Aviv University, Tel Aviv, Israel

Marcia Ramos-e-Silva, MD PhD
Head, Sector of Dermatology, Associate Professor of Dermatology,
School of Medicine and HUCFF
Universidade Federal de Rio de Janeiro, Rio de Janeiro, Brazil

Jennifer L Parish, MD
Assistant Clinical Professor of Dermatology and Cutaneous Biology,
Jefferson Medical College of Thomas Jefferson University, Philadelphia; and
Assistant Professor of Dermatology,
Tulane University School of Medicine, New Orleans, USA

informa
healthcare

New York London

First published in 2006 by Taylor & Francis, a member of the Taylor & Francis Group
This edition published in 2011 by Informa Healthcare, Telephone House, 69-77 Paul Street, London EC2A 4LQ, UK.

Simultaneously published in the USA by Informa Healthcare, 52 Vanderbilt Avenue, 7th Floor, New York, NY 10017, USA.

Informa Healthcare is a trading division of Informa UK Ltd. Registered Office: 37–41 Mortimer Street, London W1T 3JH, UK. Registered in England and Wales number 1072954.

A CIP record for this book is available from the British Library.

ISBN-13: 9781842142080

Orders may be sent to: Informa Healthcare, Sheepen Place, Colchester, Essex CO3 3LP, UK
Telephone: +44 (0)20 7017 5540
Email: CSDhealthcarebooks@informa.com
Website: http://informahealthcarebooks.com/

For corporate sales please contact: CorporateBooksIHC@informa.com
For foreign rights please contact: RightsIHC@informa.com
For reprint permissions please contact: PermissionsIHC@informa.com

Typeset by Parthenon Publishing
Printed and bound by CPI Group (UK) Ltd, Croydon, CR0 4YY
Transferred to Digital Print 2012

Contents

INFECTIONS AND INFESTATIONS

TOPOGRAPHIC DERMATOLOGY

DISEASES AND CONDITIONS OF PREGNANCY

Preface

This color *Atlas of Women's Dermatology* has been conceived to complement our book, *Women's Dermatology: From Infancy to Maturity*[1]. Although that text was illustrated with some color photography, we wanted the opportunity to provide additional pictures of skin diseases afflicting girls and women.

The word 'atlas' originally referred to the Greek god who held up 'the pillars of the universe'. In medical publishing, it has come to mean a collection of illustrations, designed with the concept that one picture is worth a thousand words[2]. With the development of the Kodachrome[TM], also termed slides or diazo-positives, enormous collections of dermatologic pictures were amassed, now augmented and even replaced with the advent of digital photography.

How then could our photographic story be told? In a previous atlas, one of the authors (LCP) utilized a morphologic format, so that diseases with manifestations on the scalp might be in that chapter and those of the leg in a separate grouping[3]. Two other atlases were organized according to disease classifications[4,5]. These three atlases also contained descriptive introductions so that the pictures would be better defined. We considered these choices but decided upon a simpler presentation with the pictures being labeled according to the illustrated skin disease and the sections being organized in the manner of the textbook chapters, where possible.

Pictures have been selected to present skin diseases in girls and women. Whereas the text-book focused on discussion of conditions that are more prevalent or different in the distaff population, we have included entities that may appear in both sexes but which we thought would be useful to illustrate. By no means should this Atlas be considered all inclusive. Some diseases may not be illustrated at all, while others might require several pictures to complete the story.

We are most appreciative of the many colleagues who have permitted us to borrow from their collections. We are also grateful to our patients who permitted their diseases to be photographed and to whom we express our thanks.

REFERENCES

1. Parish LC, Brenner S, Ramos-e-Silva M. Women's dermatology: from infancy to maturity. New York: Parthenon Publishing, 2001.

2. Kuner N, Hartschuh W. Possibilities and limits of early photography in dermatology. The 'Clinique photographique de l'hopital Saint-Louis' von 1868. Hautarzt 2003; 54: 760–4.

3. Parish LC, Kauh YC, Luscombe HA. Color atlas of difficult diagnoses in dermatology. New York: Igaku-Shoin, 1993: 1–144.

4. Parish LC, Witkowski JA, Vassileva S. Color atlas of cutaneous infections. Cambridge, MA: Blackwell Scientific, 1995: 1–176.

5. Parish LC, Sehgal VN, Buntin DM. Color atlas of sexually transmitted diseases. New York: Igaku-Shoin, 1991: 1–173.

Dermatology Lexicon Project

As a medical specialty, dermatology has the unique semantic history of overlapping and confusing diagnostic terms, eponyms, and synonyms, sometimes resulting in poor or mistaken communication and teaching. In addition, the current digital transformation of healthcare documentation and communication may even accentuate problems with terminology, rather than improve them.

In 2001, the National Institute of Arthritis and Musculoskeletal and Skin Diseases (NIAMS), National Institute of Health (NIH) National Institute of Arthritis, and the Carl J Herzog Foundation sponsored the initial development of the Dermatology Lexicon Project (DLP). Centered at the University of Rochester, the DLP has become an ongoing nationally collaborative effort of dermatologists to develop a well organized, consistent, and accurate terminology for our specialty.

The *Atlas of Women's Dermatology: From Infancy to Maturity* is the first publication to display DLP diagnostic code identifiers. The value of these codes lies not within the unique number associated with a diagnosis, but within a greater network of meaning. The codes seen in this Atlas are a subset of a much larger, detailed map of dermatologic words. Such a semantic map or classification of words strives to be a wide angled, detailed view of all of the diagnostic concepts used in the field of dermatology.

Each diagnosis in this book has a unique code. While each code represents a single diagnostic concept, a specific concept can have multiple clinical findings but only ONE meaning. The relationship between diagnoses seen within this text and other dermatologic diagnoses can be easily reviewed by searching the diagnostic term database at www.dermatologylexicon.org

Art Papier, MD
Associate Professor of Dermatology
University of Rochester School of
Medicine and Dentistry
Rochester, New York, USA

Lowell A Goldsmith, MD MPH
Professor of Dermatology
University of North Carolina School of Medicine
Chapel Hill, North Carolina, USA

This project has been funded in whole or in part with Federal funds from the National Institute of Arthritis and Musculoskeletal and Skin Diseases, National Institute of Health, Department of Health and Human Services, and with funds from the Carl J Herzog Foundation, Inc. under contract no. NO1-AR-1-2255.

Diseases of infants and children including hereditary diseases

Diseases of newborns 1

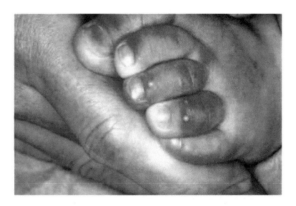

Figure 1.1 Acropustulosis, infantile. Dermatology Lexicon Project (DLP) preferred term and number: *acropustulosis of infancy 2049*. Courtesy of Dr D Wallach, Paris, France

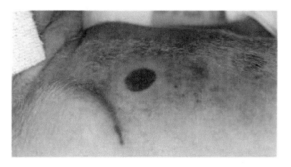

Figure 1.3 Burn, first degree due to pO_2/pCO_2 monitor. DLP ID: *first-degree burn 4045*. Courtesy of Dr D Wallach, Paris, France

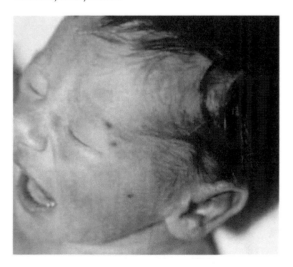

Figure 1.2 Blueberry muffin syndrome. DLP ID: *congenital cytomegalovirus infection 525*. Courtesy of Drs D Wallach and O Enjoiras, Paris, France

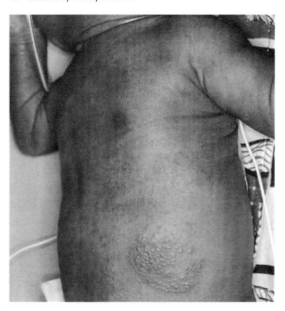

Figure 1.4 Contact dermatitis due to cardioscope probes. DLP ID: *irritant contact dermatitis 2102*. Courtesy of Dr D Wallach, Paris, France

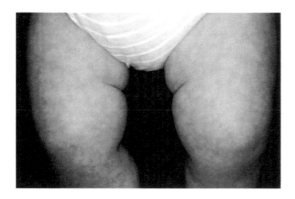

Figure 1.5 Cutis marmorata. DLP ID: *cutis marmorata 2444*. Courtesy of Dr D Wallach, Paris, France

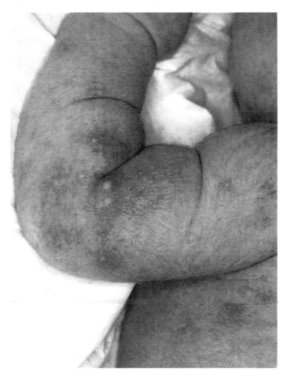

Figure 1.7 Erythema toxicum. DLP ID: *toxic erythema 4519*. Courtesy of Dr D Wallach, Paris, France

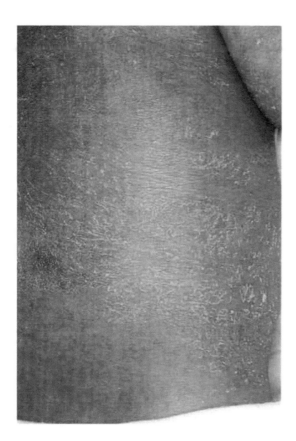

Figure 1.6 Desquamation, physiologic. DLP ID: *desquamation 4983*. Courtesy of Dr D Wallach, Paris, France

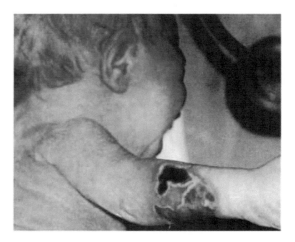

Figure 1.8 Focal dermal hypoplasia (Goltz-Gorlin syndrome) with trophic ulcer. DLP ID: *focal dermal hypoplasia 3430*. Courtesy of Dr A Metzker, Tel Aviv, Israel

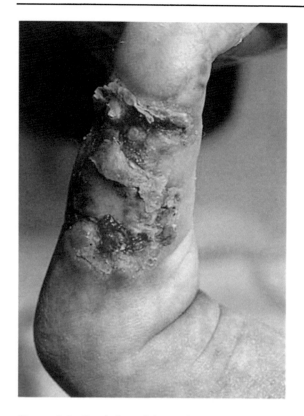

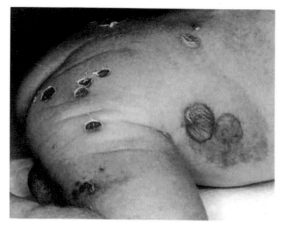

Figure 1.11 Impetigo, bullous. DLP ID: *bullous impetigo 20*. Courtesy of Dr D Wallach, Paris, France

Figure 1.9 Focal dermal hypoplasia (Goltz-Gorlin syndrome) with trophic ulcer. DLP ID: *focal dermal hypoplasia 3430*. Courtesy of Dr A Metzker, Tel Aviv, Israel

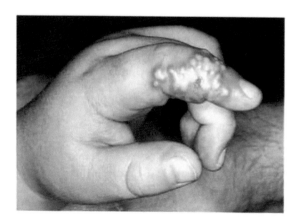

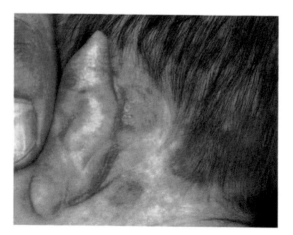

Figure 1.10 Herpes simplex infection. DLP ID: *herpes simplex virus infection 495*. Courtesy of Dr D Wallach, Paris, France

Figure 1.12 Lupus erythematosus, neonatal. DLP ID: *neonatal lupus erythematosus 1806*. Courtesy of Dr D Wallach, Paris, France

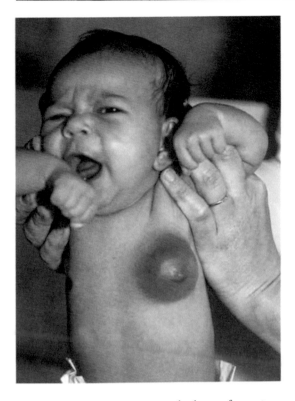

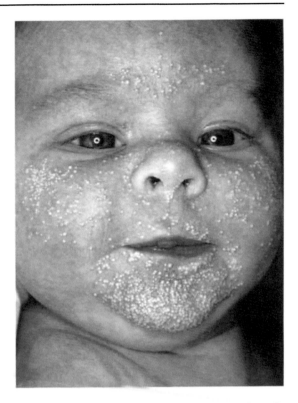

Figure 1.13 Mastitis, acute with abscess formation. DLP ID: *mastitis 6678*. Courtesy of Dr D Wallach, Paris, France

Figure 1.14 Milia, neonatal. DLP ID: *milia 843*. Courtesy of Dr D Wallach, Paris, France

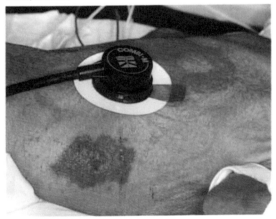

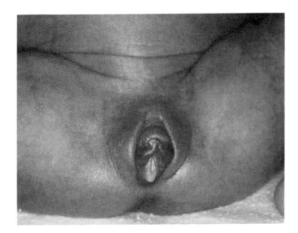

Figure 1.15 Necrosis due to prolonged contact with isopropyl alcohol-containing cleanser. DLP ID: *necrosis/ulceration of skin due to topical drug or skin preparation 5339*. Courtesy of Dr D Wallach, Paris, France

Figure 1.16 Normal vulva of a premature girl (31-week gestation). DLP ID: *normal vulva 5264*. Courtesy of Dr D Wallach, Paris, France

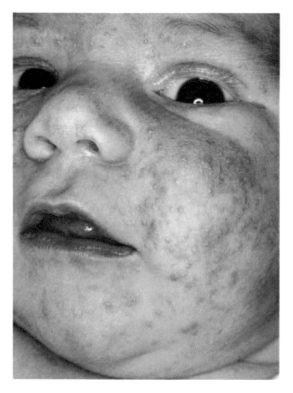

Figure 1.17 Pustulosis of the face due to *Malassezia furfur* (infantile benign cephalic pustulosis). DLP ID: *neonatal cephalic pustulosis 344*. Courtesy of Dr D Wallach, Paris, France

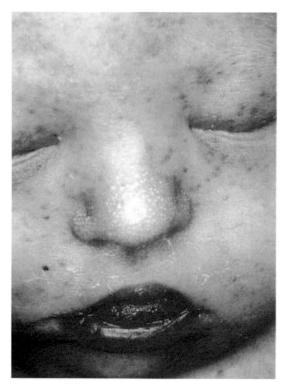

Figure 1.19 Sebaceous gland hyperplasia. DLP ID: *sebaceous hyperplasia 907*. Courtesy of Dr D Wallach, Paris, France

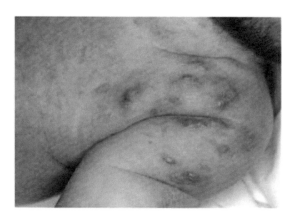

Figure 1.18 Scabies. DLP ID: *scabies infestation 463*

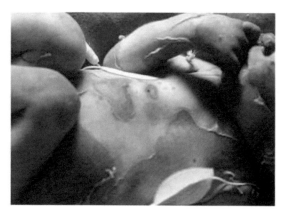

Figure 1.20 Staphylococcal scalded skin syndrome. DLP ID: *staphylococcal scalded skin syndrome 139*. Courtesy of Dr D Wallach, Paris, France

Diseases of young girls

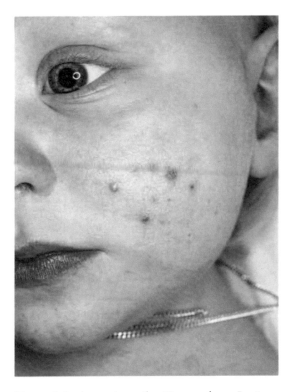

2

Figure 2.1 Acne, juvenile. Dermatology Lexicon Project (DLP) preferred term and number: *infantile acne 2289*. Courtesy of Dr D Wallach, Paris, France

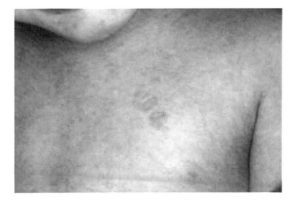

Figure 2.2 Anetoderma attributed to prematurity. DLP ID: *anetoderma of prematurity 1463*

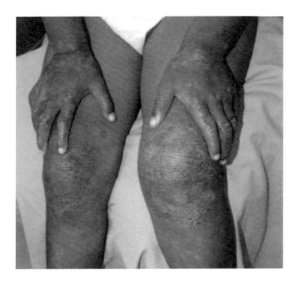

Figure 2.3 Atopic dermatitis. DLP ID: *atopic dermatitis 2100*. Courtesy of Dr NC Dlova, Durban, South Africa

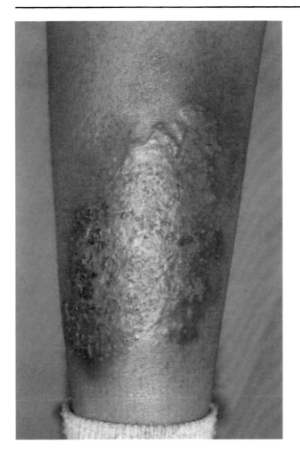

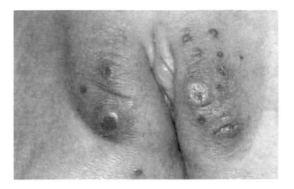

Figure 2.6 Diaper dermatitis, severe (Jacquet's dermatitis). DLP ID: *Jacquet erosive diaper dermatitis 2116*. Courtesy of Dr D Wallach, Paris, France

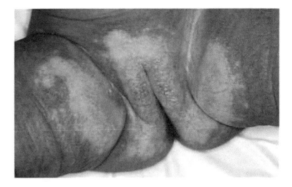

Figure 2.4 Atopic dermatitis. DLP ID: *atopic dermatitis 2100*. Courtesy of Dr NC Dlova, Durban, South Africa

Figure 2.7 Diaper dermatitis, severe, resulting in post-inflammatory hypopigmentation. DLP ID: *diaper irritant dermatitis 2125*. Courtesy of Dr D Wallach, Paris, France

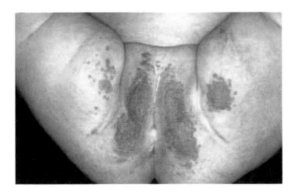

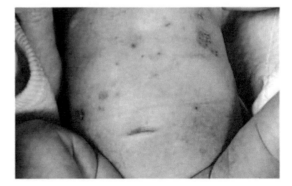

Figure 2.5 Diaper dermatitis. DLP ID: *diaper irritant dermatitis 2125*. Courtesy of Dr D Wallach, Paris, France

Figure 2.8 Histiocytosis. DLP ID: *histiocytosis 1733*

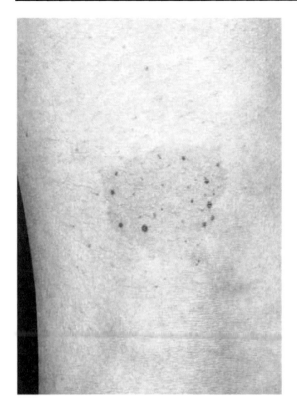

Figure 2.9 Nevus spilus. DLP ID: *nevus spilus 990*

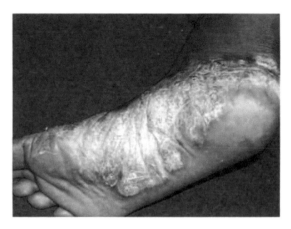

Figure 2.11 Psoriasis. DLP ID: *psoriasis 2042*

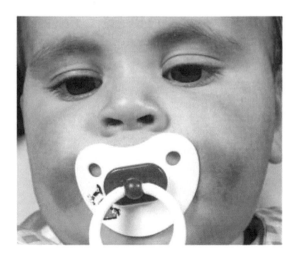

Figure 2.10 Panniculitis due to cold injury. DLP ID: *cold panniculitis 2361*

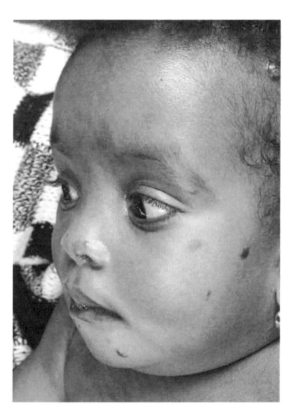

Figure 2.12 Xanthogranuloma, juvenile. DLP ID: *juvenile xanthogranuloma 4381*

Genodermatoses

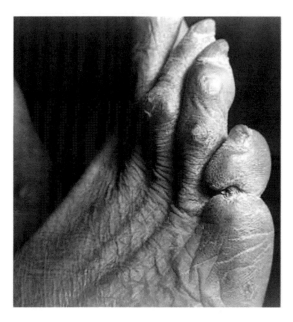

3

Figure 3.1 Ainhum. Dermatology Lexicon Project (DLP) preferred term and number: *ainhum 3404*

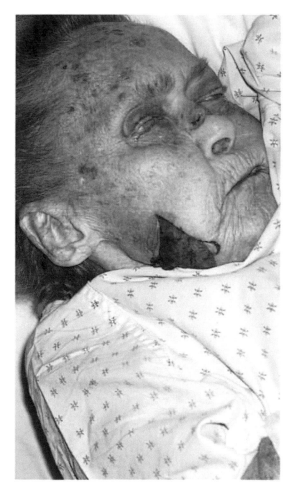

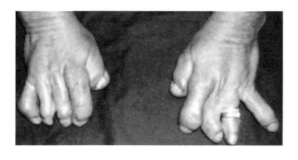

Figure 3.2 Apert syndrome (acrocephalosyndactyly). DLP ID: *Apert syndrome 3406*

Figure 3.3 Cutis laxa. DLP ID: *cutis laxa 2245*. Courtesy of Dr B Mevorach, Tel Aviv, Israel

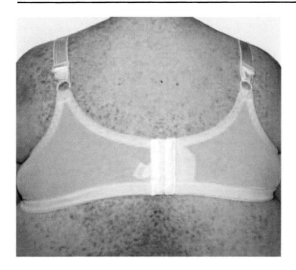

Figure 3.4 Darier's disease (keratosis follicularis). DLP ID: *Darier's disease 3078*

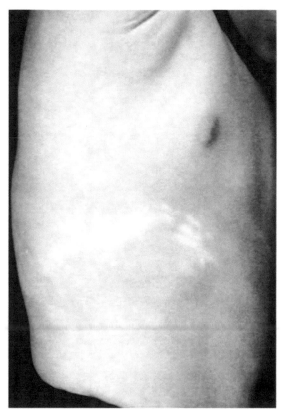

Figure 3.6 Incontinentia pigmenti achromians (hypomelanosis of Ito). DLP ID: *hypomelanosis of Ito 1035*

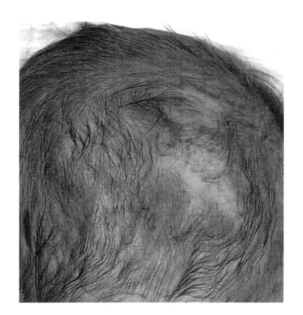

Figure 3.5 Goltz syndrome (focal dermal hypoplasia). DLP ID: *focal dermal hypoplasia 3430*

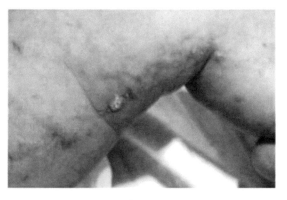

Figure 3.7 Incontinentia pigmenti (Bloch-Sulzberger syndrome). DLP ID: *incontinentia pigmenti 3239*

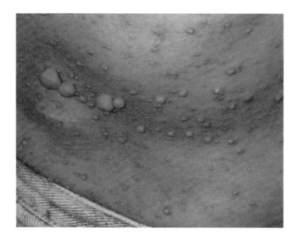

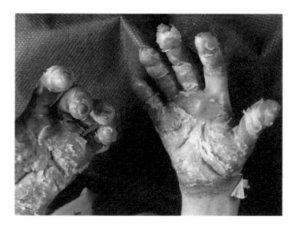

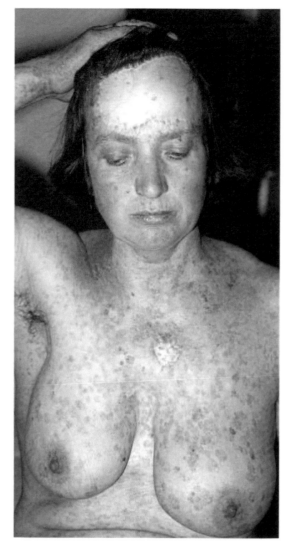

Figure 3.9 Olmstead syndrome (mutilating palmo-plantar keratoderma). DLP ID: *Olmstead syndrome 3056.* Courtesy of Dr B Mevorach, Tel Aviv, Israel

Figure 3.10 Pseudoxanthoma elasticum. DLP ID: *pseudoxanthoma elasticum 3398*

13

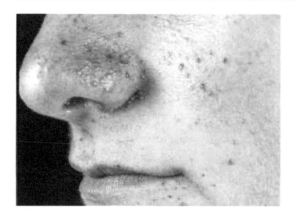

Figure 3.11 Tuberous sclerosis showing adenoma sebaceum (Bourneville's disease). DLP ID: *tuberous sclerosis 2951*. Courtesy of Dr B Mevorach, Tel Aviv, Israel

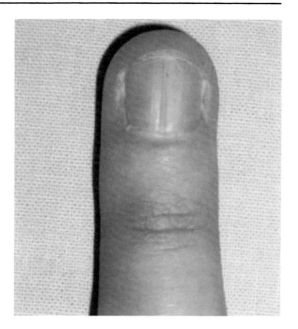

Figure 3.13 Tuberous sclerosis showing a periungual fibroma (Bourneville's disease). DLP ID: *tuberous sclerosis 2951*. Courtesy of Dr D Wallach, Paris, France

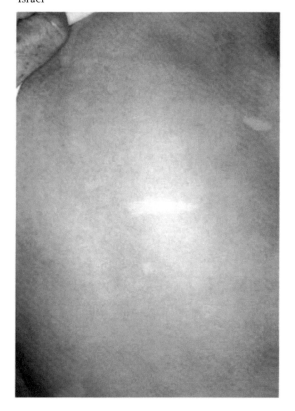

Figure 3.12 Tuberous sclerosis showing ash-leaf hypomelanotic macule (Bourneville's disease). DLP ID: *tuberous sclerosis 2951*. Courtesy of Dr D Wallach, Paris, France

Diseases of
skin structure – non-hereditary

Disorders of the sebaceous, apocrine, and eccrine glands

4

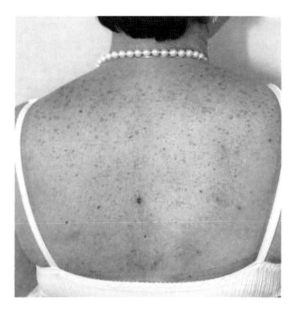

Figure 4.1 Acne aggravated by oral steroids. Dermatology Lexicon Project (DLP) preferred term and number: *steroid induced acne 2295*

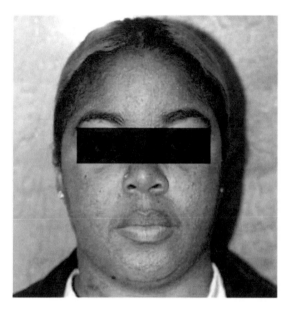

Figure 4.2 Acne aggravated by Vaseline®. DLP ID: *pomade acne 2300*

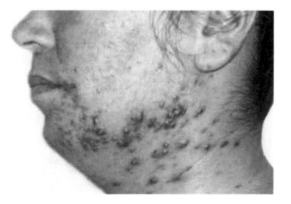

Figure 4.3 Acne conglobata. DLP ID: *acne conglobata 2318*

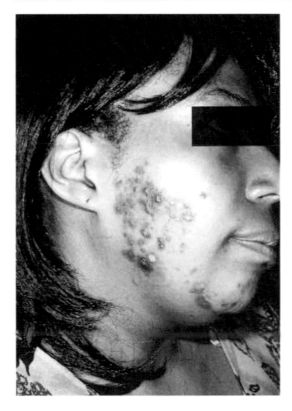

Figure 4.4 Acne excoriée de jeune fille. DLP ID: *acne excoriee 653*

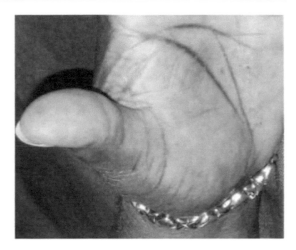

Figure 4.6 Dyshidrosis. DLP ID: *dyshidrotic dermatitis 2107*

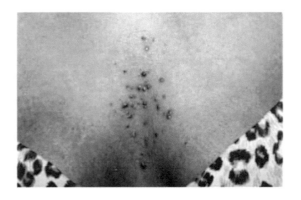

Figure 4.5 Acne keloidalis. DLP ID: *acne keloidalis 2321*

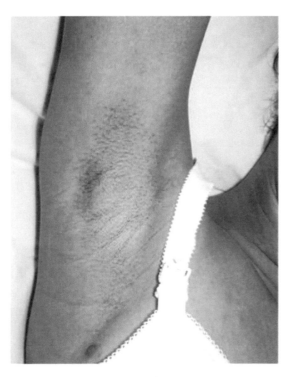

Figure 4.7 Fox-Fordyce disease. DLP ID: *Fox-Fordyce disease 2348*

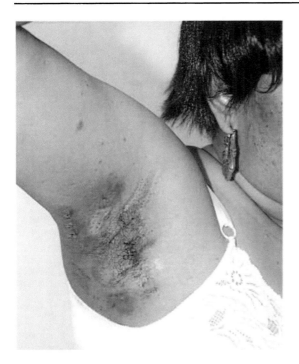

Figure 4.8 Hidradenitis suppurativa in the axilla. DLP ID: *hidradenitis suppurativa 2317*

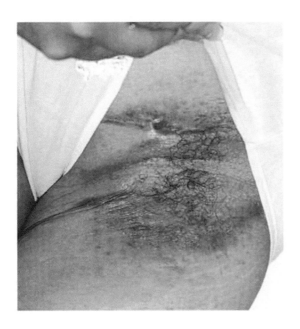

Figure 4.9 Hidradenitis suppurativa in the inguinal area. DLP ID: *hidradenitis suppurativa 2317*

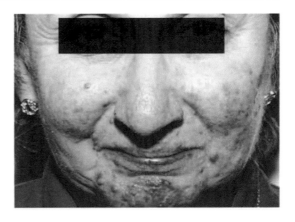

Figure 4.10 Perioral dermatitis. DLP ID: *perioral dermatitis 2313*

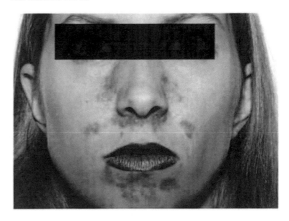

Figure 4.11 Rosacea. DLP ID: *rosacea 2283*

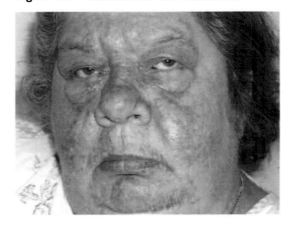

Figure 4.12 Rosacea with rhinophyma in a woman with hyperandrogenism. DLP ID: *rosacea 2283*

Disorders of the nails 5

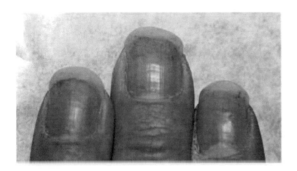

Figure 5.1 Alopecia areata with Scotch plaiding. Dermatology Lexicon Project (DLP) preferred term and number: *alopecia areata 1841*

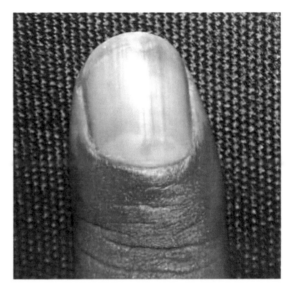

Figure 5.3 Glomangioma. DLP ID: *glomangioma 1468*. Courtesy of Dr A d'Acri, Rio de Janeiro, Brazil

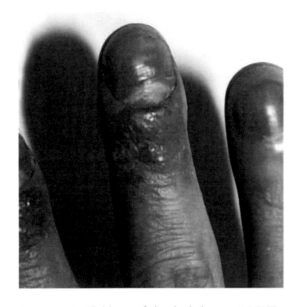

Figure 5.2 Clubbing of distal phalanges. DLP ID: *idiopathic clubbing of fingers 4494*

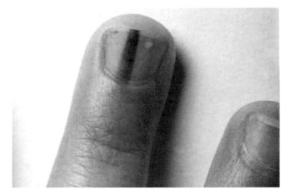

Figure 5.4 Melanonychia, benign, longitudinal due to nevus, pigmented. DLP ID: *melanonychia striata 1082*

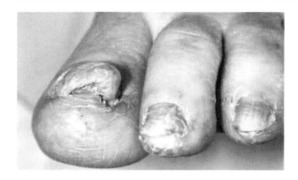

Figure 5.5 Onychomycosis. DLP ID: *onychomycosis 4935*

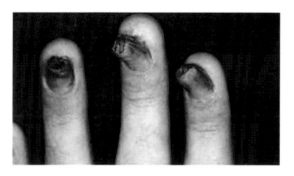

Figure 5.6 Pachyonychia congenita. DLP ID: *pachyonychia congenita 3270*

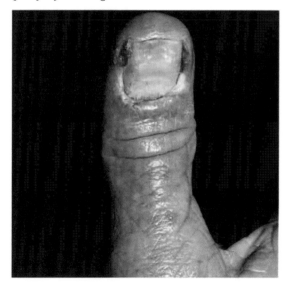

Figure 5.7 Paronychia due to *Candida albicans*. DLP ID: *paronychia canididiasis 362*

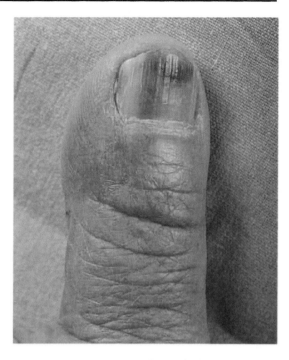

Figure 5.8 Pigmentation due to hydroxyurea therapy for polycythemia vera. DLP ID: *nail pigment, drug induced 4222*

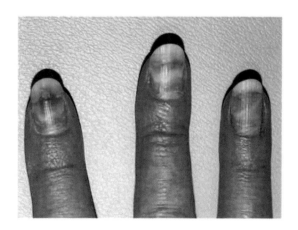

Figure 5.9 Pseudomonas nail infection. DLP ID: *pseudomonas nail infection 4816*

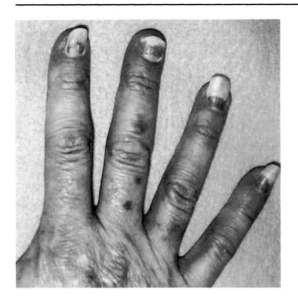

Figure 5.10 Psoriatic nails. DLP ID: *psoriasis of the nails 4751*

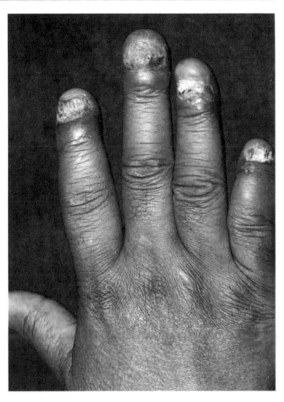

Figure 5.12 Sarcoidosis. DLP ID: *sarcoidosis 2203*

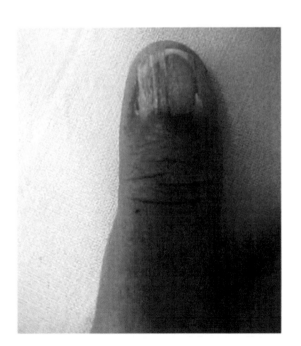

Figure 5.11 Pterygium. DLP ID: *pterygium 4799.* Courtesy of Dr T Cestari, Porto Alegre, Brazil

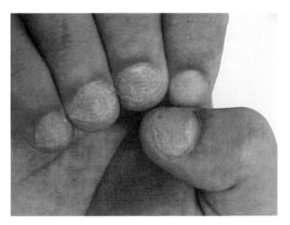

Figure 5.13 Trachyonychia. DLP ID: *trachyonychia 3928*

Disorders of the hair and the scalp 6

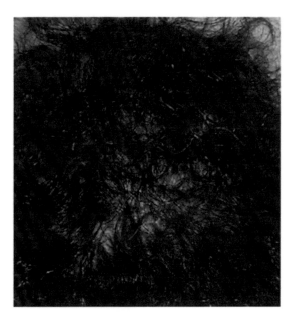

Figure 6.1 Alopecia androgenic. Dermatology Lexicon Project (DLP) preferred term and number: *patterned hair loss 3737*

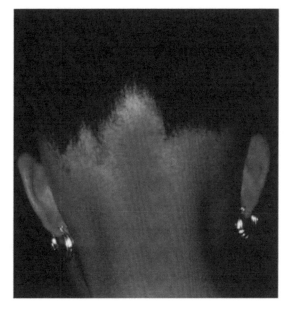

Figure 6.2 Alopecia areata. DLP ID: *alopecia areata 1841*

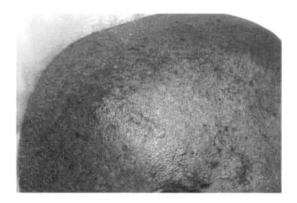

Figure 6.3 Alopecia due to hot combs. DLP ID: *hot comb alopecia 4663*

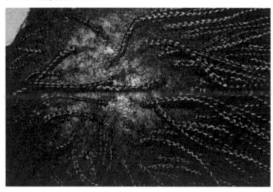

Figure 6.4 Alopecia due to traction from braiding. DLP ID: *traction alopecia 3860*

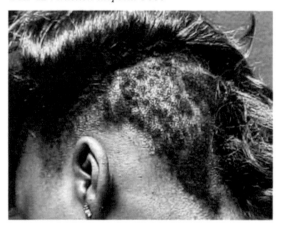

Figure 6.5 Alopecia due to traction from curlers. DLP ID: *traction alopecia 3860*. Courtesy of Dr D Van Neste, Tournai, Belgium

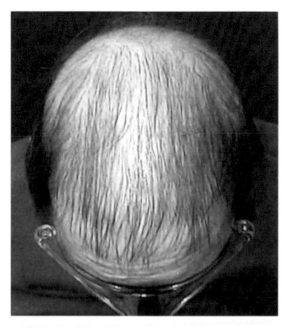

Figure 6.6 Alopecia, permanent following chemotherapy for breast cancer with docetaxel. DLP ID: *alopecia (unclassified) 4950*. Courtesy of Dr D Van Neste, Tournai, Belgium

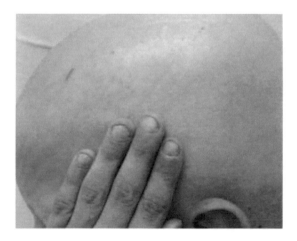

Figure 6.7 Alopecia totalis with Scotch plaiding of nails. DLP ID: *alopecia totalis 3782*

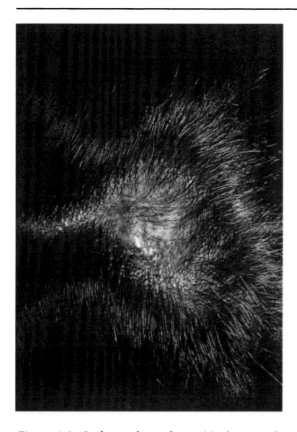

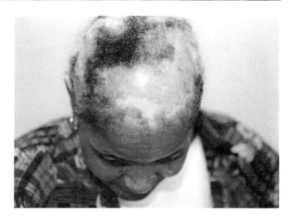

Figure 6.10 Lupus erythematosus, discoid with alopecia. DLP ID: *discoid lupus erythematosus, 1803*

Figure 6.8 Lichen planopilaris (Graham-Little syndrome). DLP ID: *lichen planopilaris 2152*

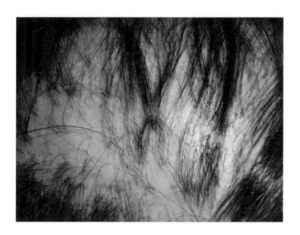

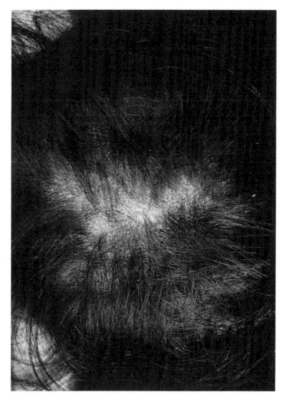

Figure 6.9 Lichen planopilaris (Graham-Little syndrome). DLP ID: *lichen planopilaris (Graham-Little syndrome) 2152*. Courtesy of Drs C Sodre and G Munhoz-da-Fontoura, Rio de Janeiro, Brazil

Figure 6.11 Lupus erythematosus, systemic with alopecia. DLP ID: *systemic lupus erythematosus, 1808*

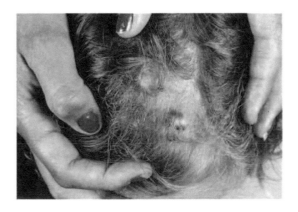

Figure 6.12 Nevus, woolly hair. DLP ID: *woolly hair nevus 4525*

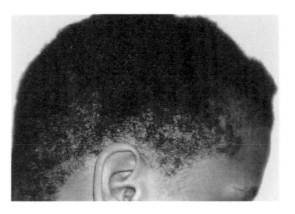

Figure 6.13 Ophiasis. DLP ID: *ophiasis 1854*

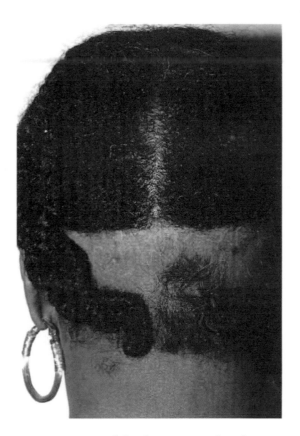

Figure 6.14 Perifolliculitis capitis abscedens et suffodiens (dissecting cellulitis of the scalp). DLP ID: *dissecting cellulitis of the scalp 2319*

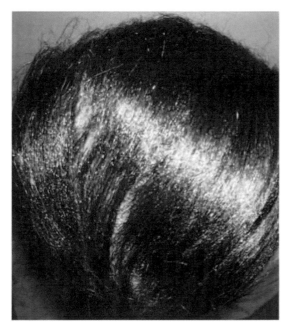

Figure 6.15 Pseudopelade of Brocq. DLP ID: *pseudopelade of Brocq 5266*

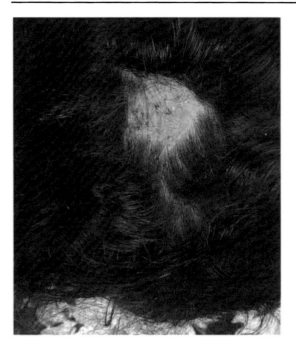

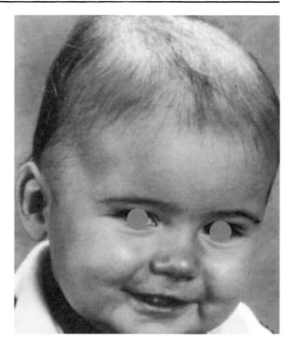

Figure 6.16 Tinea capitis in an adult due to *Microsporum canis*. DLP ID: *tinea capitis 321*. Courtesy of Dr D Van Neste, Tournai, Belgium

Figure 6.17 Trichothiodystrophy. DLP ID: *trichothiodystrophy 3763*. Courtesy of Dr D Van Neste, Tournai, Belgium

Other diseases

Papulosquamous diseases

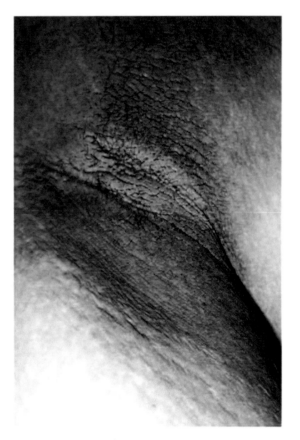

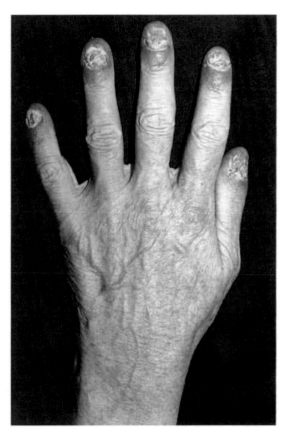

Figure 7.1 Acanthosis nigricans. Dermatology Lexicon Project (DLP) preferred term and number: *acanthosis nigricans 2797*

Figure 7.2 Acrodermatitis continua of Hallopeau. DLP ID: *acrodermatitis continua 2050*

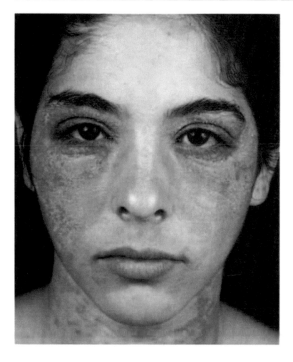

Figure 7.3 Atopic dermatitis. DLP ID: *atopic dermatitis 2100*

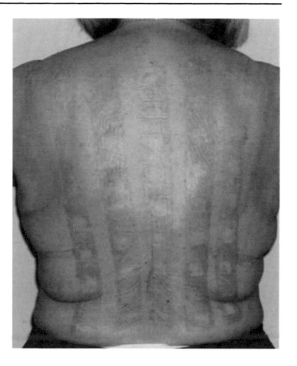

Figure 7.5 Contact dermatitis due to adhesive patches (also shows two positive patch test reactions). DLP ID: *allergic contact dermatitis 2101*

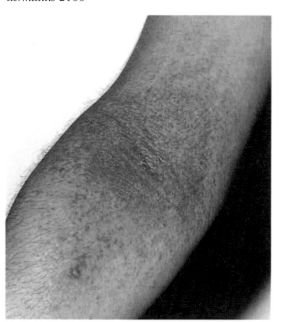

Figure 7.4 Atopic dermatitis. DLP ID: *atopic dermatitis 2100*

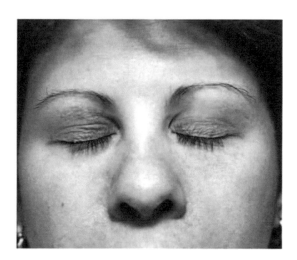

Figure 7.6 Contact dermatitis due to eye cream. DLP ID: *allergic contact dermatitis 2101*

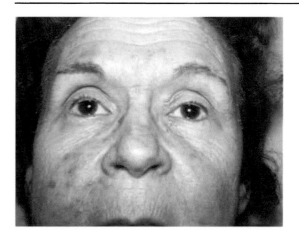

Figure 7.7 Contact dermatitis due to hair dye. DLP ID: *allergic contact dermatitis 2101*

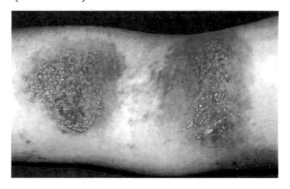

Figure 7.8 Contact dermatitis due to rivet of jeans (nickel-based). DLP ID: *nickel dermatitis 4077*

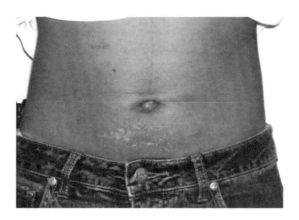

Figure 7.9 Contact dermatitis – rhus dermatitis. DLP ID: *allergic contact dermatitis due to plant 3790*

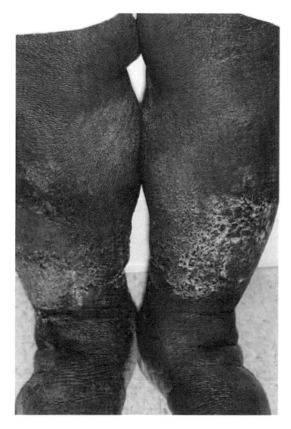

Figure 7.10 Elephantiasis. DLP ID: *elephantiasis verrucosa nostra 2486*

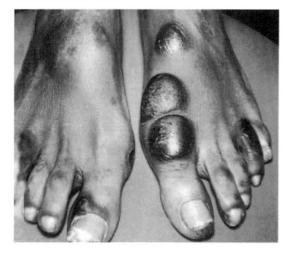

Figure 7.11 Erythema elevatum diutinum. DLP ID: *erythema elevatum diutinum 2013*

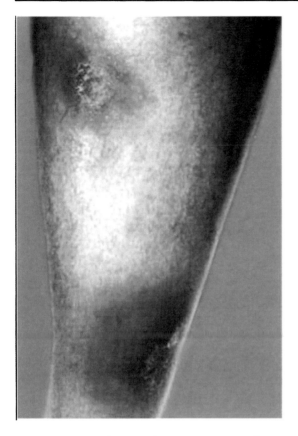

Figure 7.12 Erythema nodosum. DLP ID: *erythema nodosum 2353*

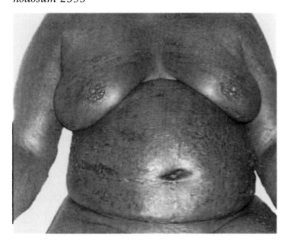

Figure 7.13 Exfoliative erythroderma due to chronic atopic dermatitis. DLP ID: *exfoliative dermatitis 2118*

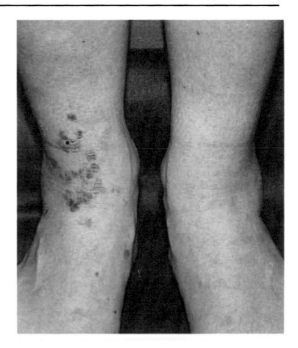

Figure 7.14 Granuloma annulare. DLP ID: *granuloma annulare 2200*

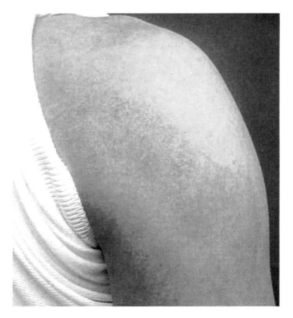

Figure 7.15 Keratosis pilaris. DLP ID: *keratosis pilaris 2324*

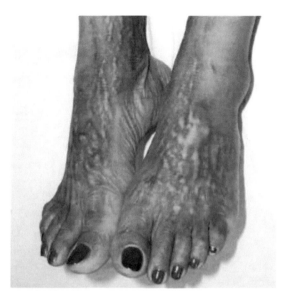

Figure 7.16 Lichen amyloidosis. DLP ID: *lichen amyloidosis 2623*. Courtesy of Dr G Munhoz-da-Fontoura, Rio de Janeiro, Brazil

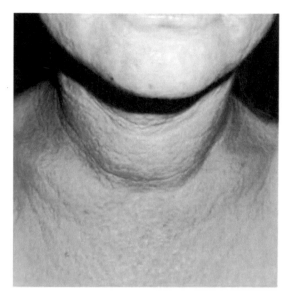

Figure 7.18 Lipoid proteinosis (Urbach-Wiethe syndrome). DLP ID: *lipoid proteinosis 2642*. Courtesy of Drs J Brack and Dr G Munhoz-da-Fontoura, Rio de Janeiro, Brazil

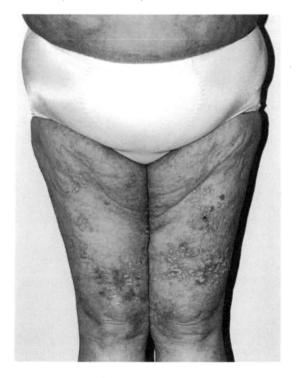

Figure 7.17 Lichen planus. DLP ID: *lichen planus 4843*

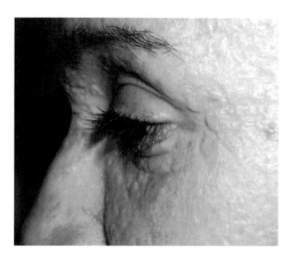

Figure 7.19 Lipoid proteinosis (Urbach-Wiethe syndrome). DLP ID: *lipoid proteinosis 2642*. Courtesy of Drs J Brack and Dr G Munhoz-da-Fontoura, Rio de Janeiro, Brazil

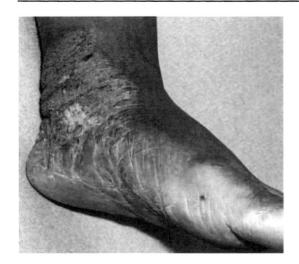

Figure 7.20 Neurodermatitis. DLP ID: *neurodermatitis 4790*

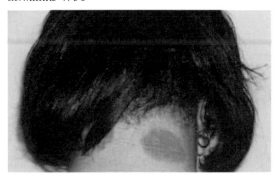

Figure 7.21 Nummular dermatitis. DLP ID: *nummular dermatitis 2104*

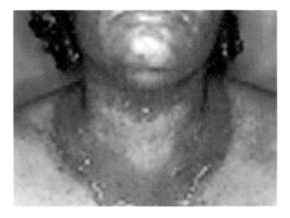

Figure 7.22 Pellagra. DLP ID: *pellagra 2740*

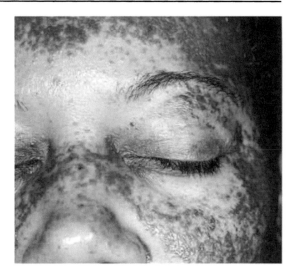

Figure 7.23 Photocontact dermatitis due to celery (phytophotodermatitis). DLP ID: *phytophotodermatitis 2123*

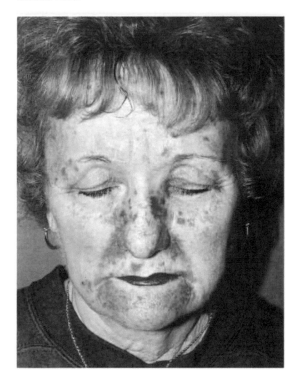

Figure 7.24 Photocontact dermatitis due to 5-fluorouracil. DLP ID: *photoallergic reaction, drug induced 1903*

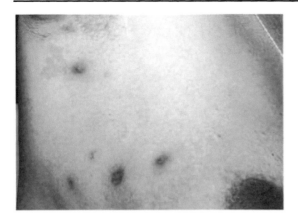

Figure 7.25 Pityriasis lichenoides et varioliformis acuta (PLEVA) (Mucha-Habermann disease). DLP ID: *parapsoriasis lichenoides et varioliformis acuta (PLEVA) 2023*

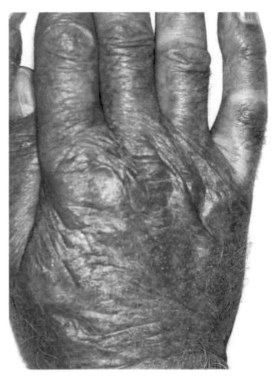

Figure 7.27 Pityriasis rubra pilaris. DLP ID: *pityriasis rubra pilaris 2043*

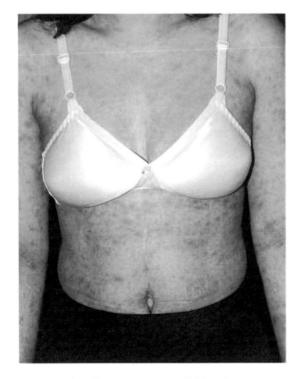

Figure 7.26 Pityriasis rosea. DLP ID: *pityriasis rosea 2058*

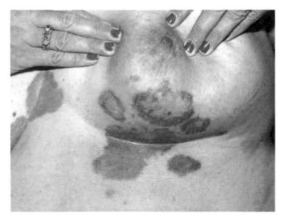

Figure 7.28 Psoriasis. DLP ID: *psoriasis 2042*

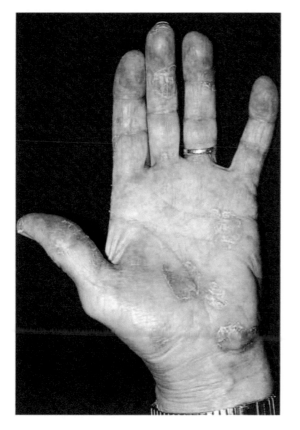

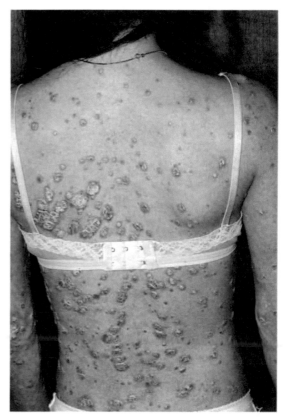

Figure 7.29 Psoriasis. DLP ID: *psoriasis 2042*

Figure 7.30 Psoriasis. DLP ID: *psoriasis 2042*

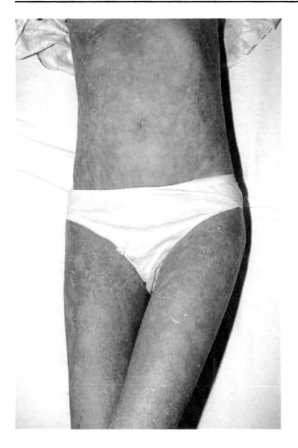

Figure 7.31 Psoriasis. DLP ID: *psoriasis 2042*

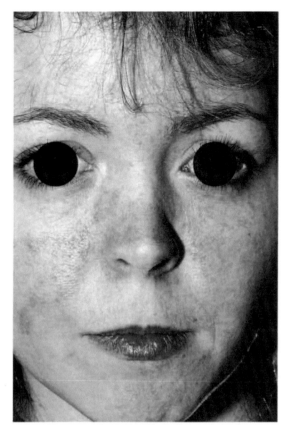

Figure 7.33 Seborrheic dermatitis. DLP ID: *seborrheic dermatitis 2105*

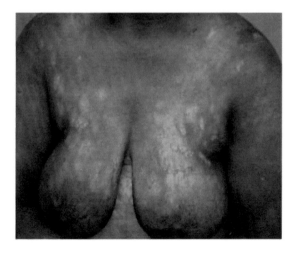

Figure 7.32 Psoriasis. DLP ID: *psoriasis 2042*. Courtesy of Dr NC Dlova, Durban, South Africa

Diseases of pigment changes 8

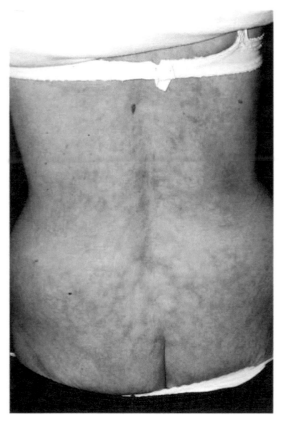

Figure 8.1 Erythema ab igne. Dermatology Lexicon Project (DLP) preferred term and number: *erythema ab igne 4048*

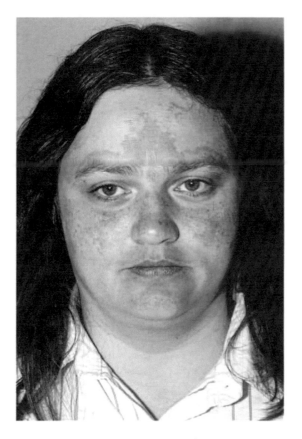

Figure 8.2 Melasma. DLP ID: *melasma 4200*

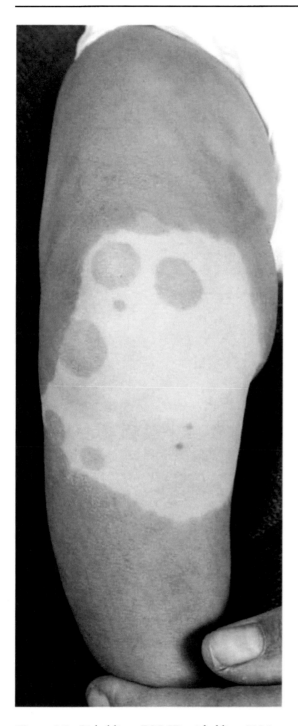

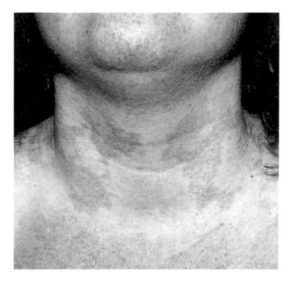

Figure 8.4 Poikiloderma of Civatte. DLP ID: *poikiloderma of Civatte 4444*

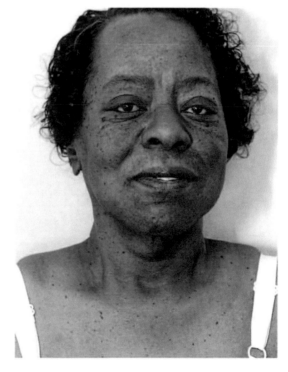

Figure 8.3 Piebaldism. DLP ID: *piebaldism 3184*

Figure 8.5 Post-inflammatory hyperpigmentation. DLP ID: *post-inflammatory hyperpigmentation 5261*

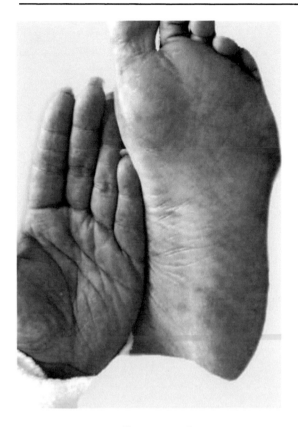

Figure 8.6 Post-inflammatory hyperpigmentation due to doxorubicin therapy for cancer. DLP ID: *hyperpigmentation, drug induced 4942*

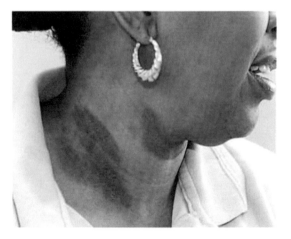

Figure 8.7 Riehl's melanosis (berloque dermatitis due to partner's cologne). DLP ID: *pigmented contact dermatitis 4455*

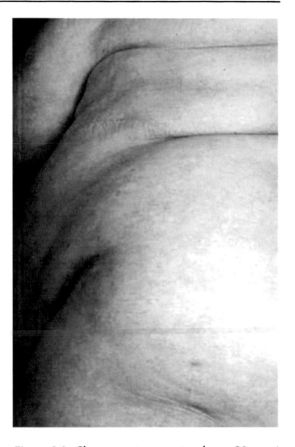

Figure 8.8 Slate gray pigmentation due to 20 years' ingestion of minocycline. DLP ID: *hyperpigmentation, drug induced 4942*

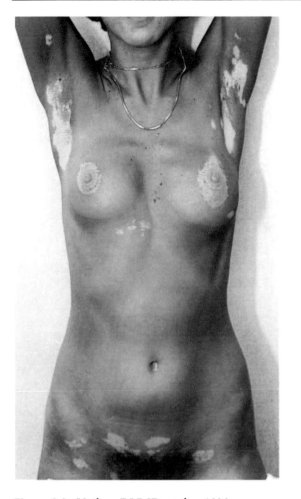

Figure 8.9 Vitiligo. DLP ID: *vitiligo 1839*

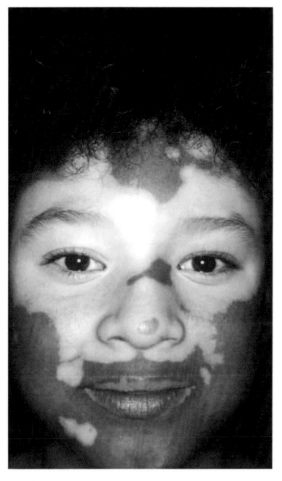

Figure 8.10 Vitiligo. DLP ID: *vitiligo 1839*

Vesicular and bullous diseases 9

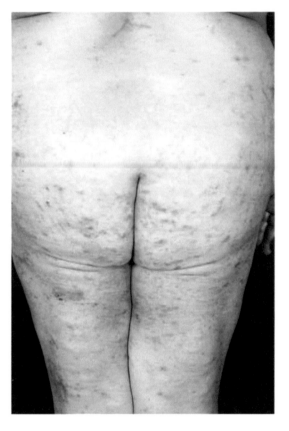

Figure 9.1 Dermatitis herpetiformis (Duhring's disease). Dermatology Lexicon Project (DLP) preferred term and number: *dermatitis herpetiformis 1764*

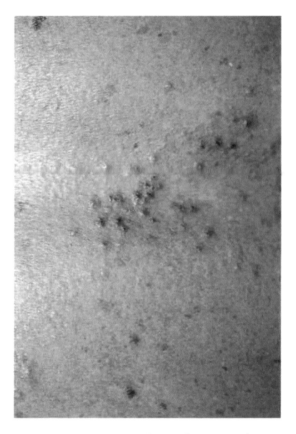

Figure 9.2 Dermatitis herpetiformis (Duhring's disease). DLP ID: *dermatitis herpetiformis 1764*

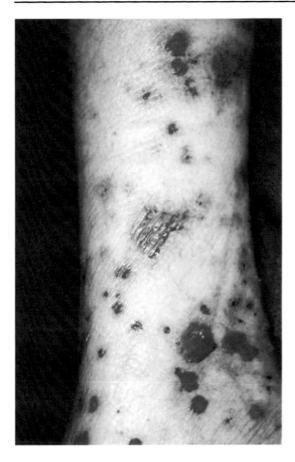

Figure 9.3 Diabetic bulla. DLP ID: *bullosis diabeticorum 2799*. Courtesy of Dr G Lestringent, Abu Dahbi, United Arab Emirates

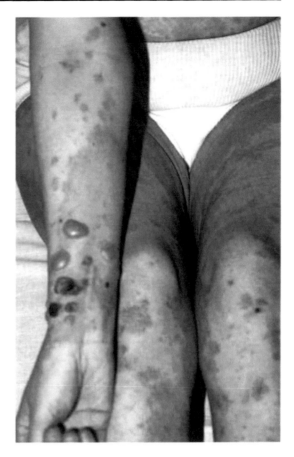

Figure 9.5 Pemphigoid, bullous. DLP ID: *pemphigoid, bullous 1760*

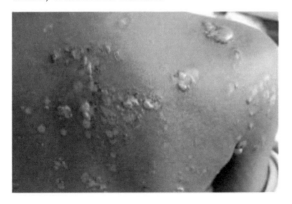

Figure 9.4 Linear IgA bullous dermatosis. DLP ID: *linear bullous dermatosis 1765*. Courtesy of Dr S Vassileva, Sofia, Bulgaria

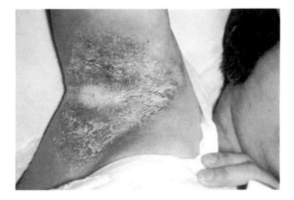

Figure 9.6 Pemphigus, benign familial chronic (Hailey–Hailey disease). DLP ID: *Hailey–Hailey disease 3503*

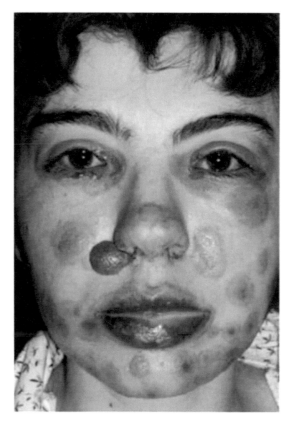

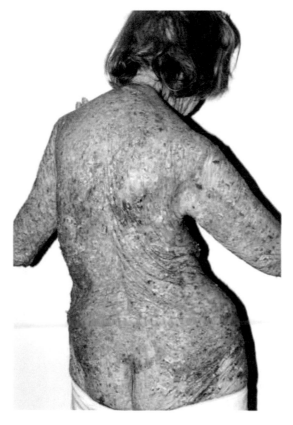

Figure 9.7 Pemphigus erythematosus (Senear Usher syndrome). DLP ID: *pemphigus erythematosus 1751*. Courtesy of Dr I Botev, Sofia, Bulgaria

Figure 9.8 Pemphigus foliaceus. DLP ID: *pemphigus foliaceus 1750*

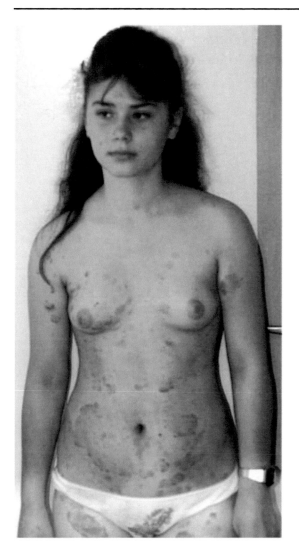

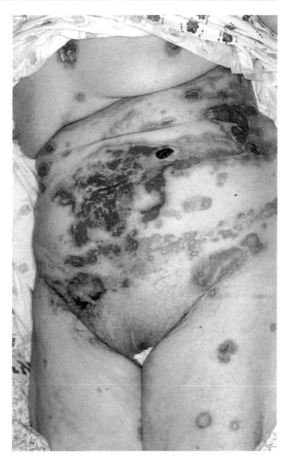

Figure 9.10 Pemphigus vulgaris. DLP ID: *pemphigus vulgaris 1748*

Figure 9.9 Pemphigus herpetiformis. DLP ID: *pemphigus herpetiformis 1755*

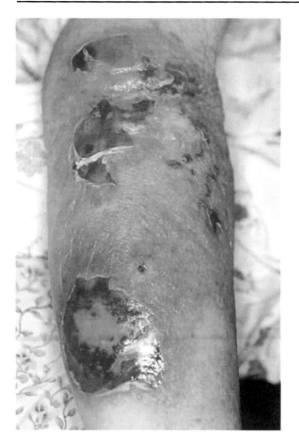

Figure 9.11 Pemphigus vulgaris. DLP ID: *pemphigus vulgaris 1748*

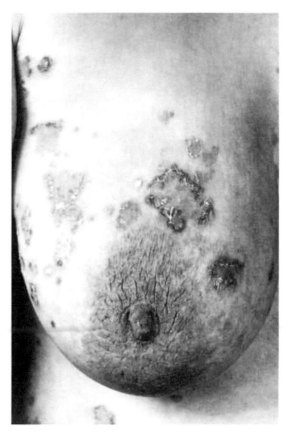

Figure 9.13 Subcorneal pustulosis of Sneddon and Wilkinson. DLP ID: *subcorneal pustular dermatosis 1769*

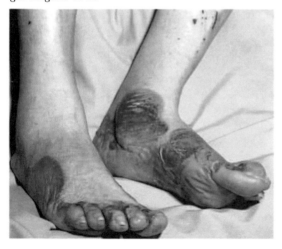

Figure 9.12 Pemphigus vulgaris. DLP ID: *pemphigus vulgaris 1748*

Connective tissue diseases 10

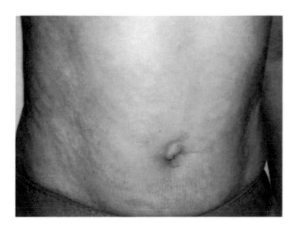

Figure 10.1 Anetoderma following secondary syphilis. Dermatology Lexicon Project (DLP) preferred term and number: *anetoderma 2241*. Courtesy of Drs N Fernandes and G Munhoz-da-Fontoura, Rio de Janeiro, Brazil

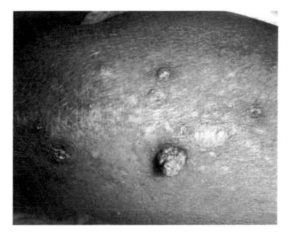

Figure 10.3 Calcinosis cutis. DLP ID: *calcinosis cutis 2679*

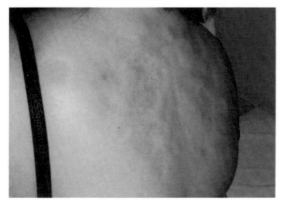

Figure 10.2 Atrophoderma of Pasini and Pierini. DLP ID: *atrophoderma of Pasini and Pierini 1823*. Courtesy of Dr G Munhoz-da-Fontoura, Rio de Janeiro, Brazil

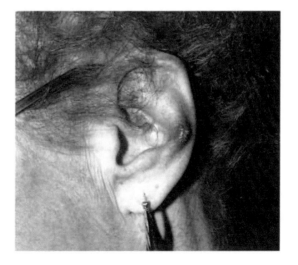

Figure 10.4 Chondrodermatitis nodularis helicis. DLP ID: *chondrodermatitis nodularis helicis 1201*

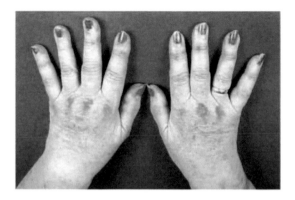

Figure 10.5 Dermatomyositis. DLP ID: *dermato-myositis 1796*

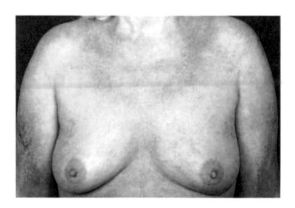

Figure 10.6 Dermatomyositis. DLP ID: *dermato-myositis 1796*

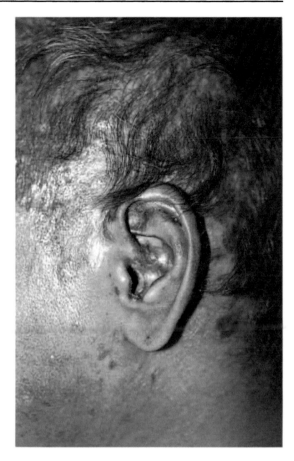

Figure 10.8 Lupus erythematosus, discoid. DLP ID: *discoid lupus erythematosus 1803*

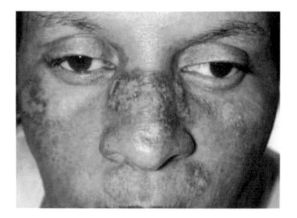

Figure 10.7 Lupus erythematosus, discoid. DLP ID: *lupus erythematosus discoid 1803*

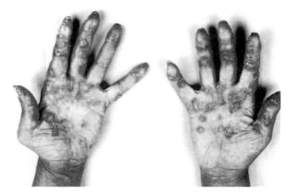

Figure 10.9 Lupus erythematosus, systemic. DLP ID: *systemic lupus erythematosus 1808*

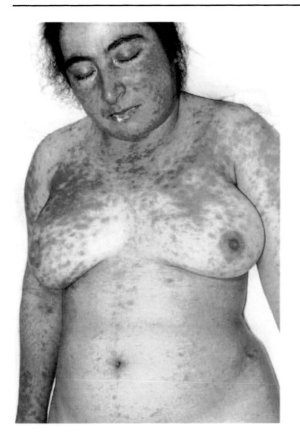

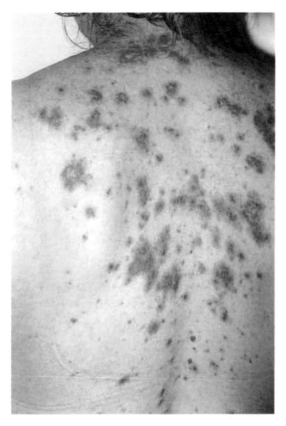

Figure 10.10 Lupus erythematosus, systemic. DLP ID: *systemic lupus erythematosus 1808*

Figure 10.11 Lupus erythematosus, systemic associated with lung cancer. DLP ID: *systemic lupus erythematosus 1808*

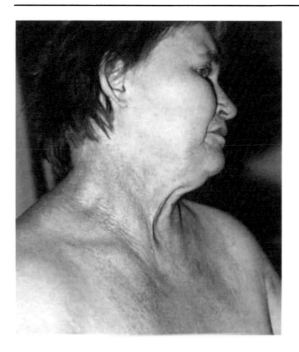

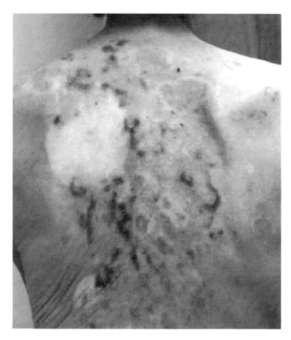

Figure 10.12 Pseudoxanthoma elasticum. DLP ID: *pseudoxanthoma elasticum 3398*

Figure 10.14 Scleroderma. DLP ID: *scleroderma 1795*

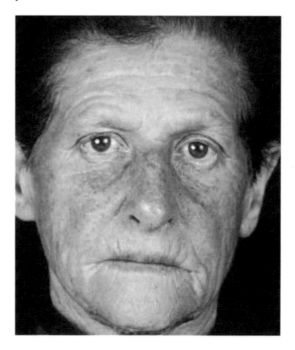

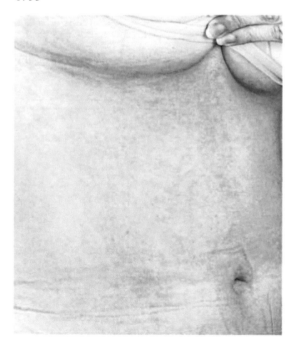

Figure 10.13 Scleroderma. DLP ID: *scleroderma 1795*

Figure 10.15 Scleroderma, morphea. DLP ID: *morphea 1821*

Vascular diseases

11

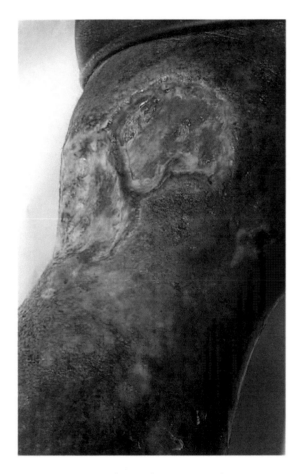

Figure 11.1 Decubitus ulcer. Dermatology Lexicon Project (DLP) preferred term and number: *decubitus ulcer 3853*

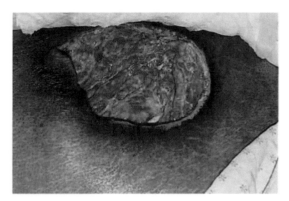

Figure 11.2 Decubitus ulcer. DLP ID: *decubitus ulcer 3853*

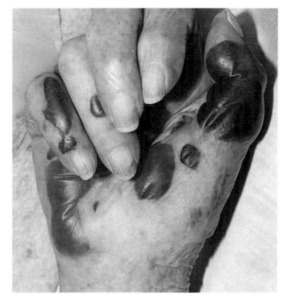

Figure 11.3 Decubitus ulcer – bullous. DLP ID: *decubitus ulcer 3853*

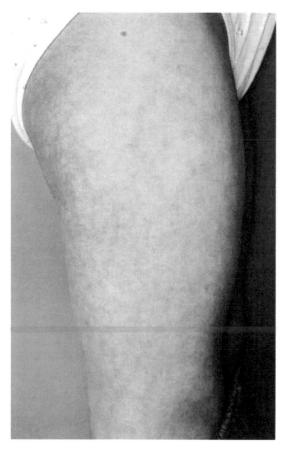

Figure 11.4 Livedo reticularis. DLP ID: *livedo reticularis 2441*

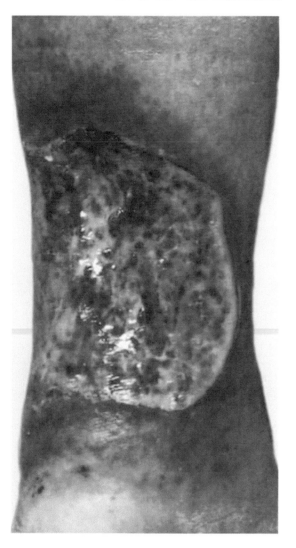

Figure 11.5 Pyoderma gangrenosum. DLP ID: *pyoderma gangrenosum 2164*

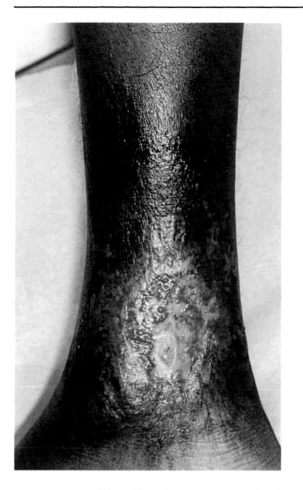

Figure 11.6 Sickle cell leg ulcer. DLP ID: *sickle cell ulcer 6695*

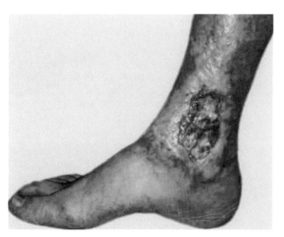

Figure 11.8 Stasis dermatitis. DLP ID: *stasis dermatitis 2109*

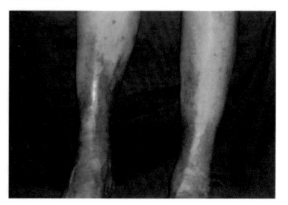

Figure 11.7 Stasis dermatitis. DLP ID: *stasis dermatitis 2109*

Figure 11.9 Stasis ulcer with stasis dermatitis. DLP ID: *stasis ulcer 2514*

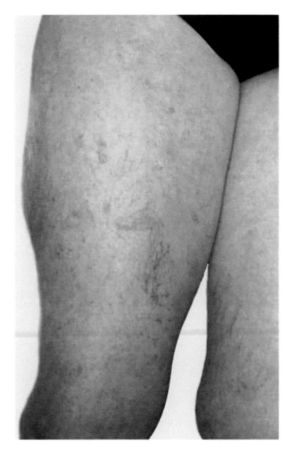

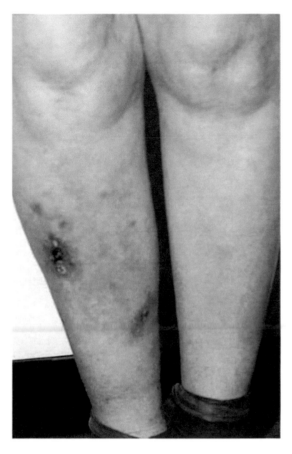

Figure 11.10 Varicosities and telangiectasias. DLP ID: *varicosities 2539*

Figure 11.11 Vasculitis, necrotizing. DLP ID: *necrotizing vasculitis 2858*

Cutaneous tumors

12

BENIGN AND PREMALIGNANT

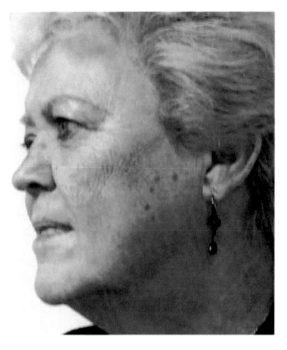

Figure 12.1 Actinic damage with seborrheic keratoses. Dermatology Lexicon Project (DLP) preferred term and number: *actinic damage 6697*

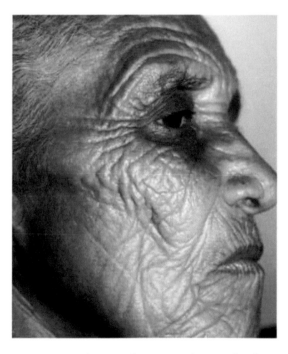

Figure 12.2 Actinic damage without seborrheic keratoses. DLP ID: *actinic damage 6697*. Courtesy of Dr T Cestari, Porto Alegre, Brazil

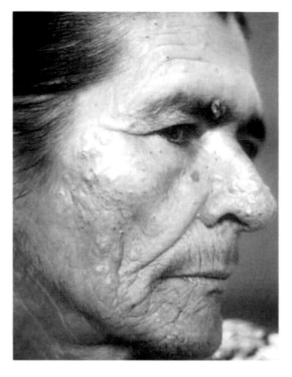

Figure 12.3 Actinic keratoses with nodular elastosis, cysts, and comedones (Favre-Racouchot syndrome). DLP ID: *actinic keratosis 775*. Courtesy of Dr T Cestari, Porto Alegre, Brazil

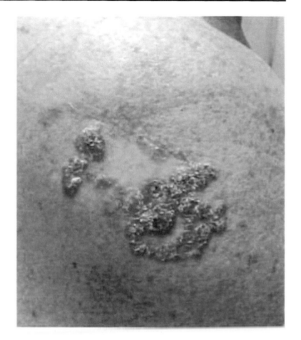

Figure 12.5 Bowen's disease (squamous cell carcinoma intraepidermal). DLP ID: *squamous cell carcinoma in-situ 788*

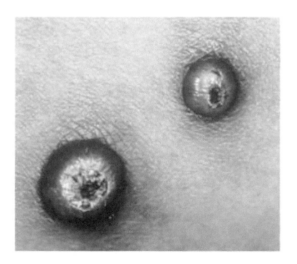

Figure 12.4 Angiolymphoid hyperplasia. DLP ID: *angiolymphoid hyperplasia with eosinophilia 1423*

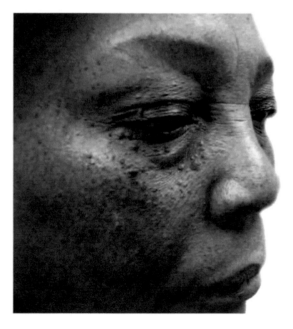

Figure 12.6 Dermatosis papulosa nigrans. DLP ID: *dermatosis papulosa nigra 754*

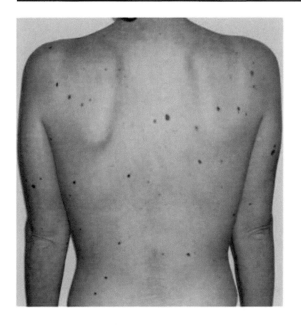

Figure 12.7 Dysplastic nevus syndrome. DLP ID: *familial atypical mole-melanoma syndrome 3229*

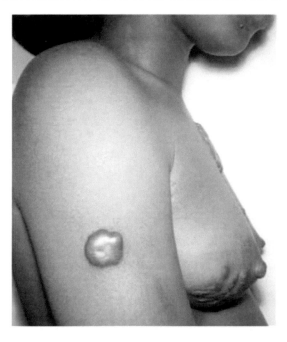

Figure 12.9 Keloid. DLP ID: *keloid 1264*

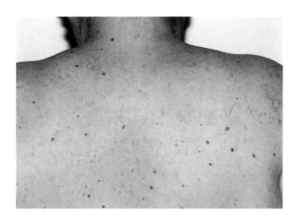

Figure 12.8 Cherry angioma. DLP ID: *cherry angioma 1433*

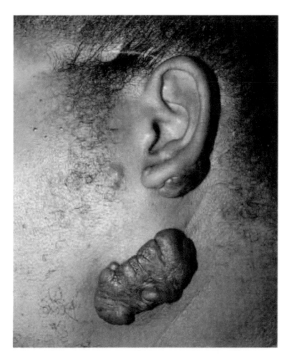

Figure 12.10 Keloid. DLP ID: *keloid 1264*

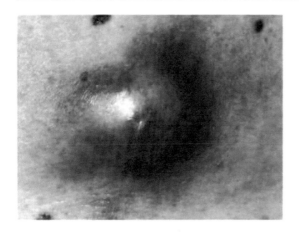

Figure 12.11 Keratinous cyst, infected. DLP ID: *epidermoid cyst 853*

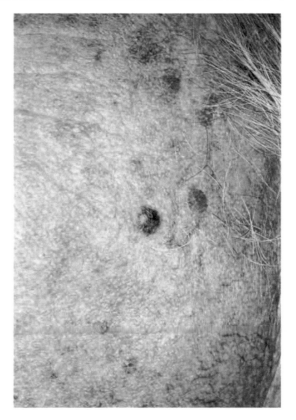

Figure 12.13 Nevus, blue of Jadassohn. DLP ID: *blue nevus 1036*

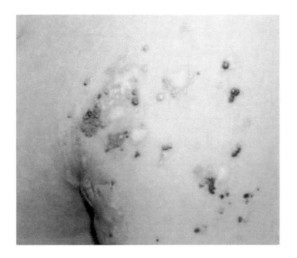

Figure 12.12 Lymphangioma circumscriptum. DLP ID: *lymphangioma circumscriptum 1477.* Courtesy of Dr I Botev, Sofia, Bulgaria

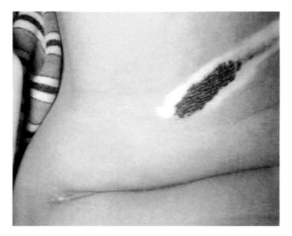

Figure 12.14 Nevus, halo of Sutton. DLP ID: *halo nevus 1014*

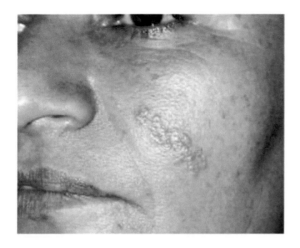

Figure 12.15 Nevus, sebaceous of Jadassohn. DLP ID: *benign sebaceous gland tumor 903*

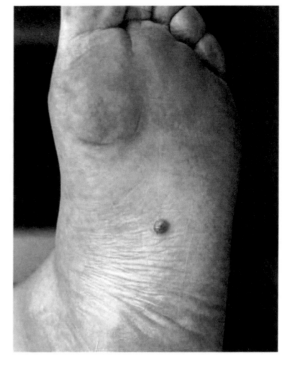

Figure 12.17 Poroma, eccrine. DLP ID: *eccrine poroma 935*

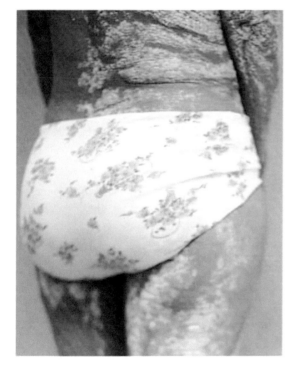

Figure 12.16 Nevus unis lateralis. DLP ID: *nevus unis lateralis 748*

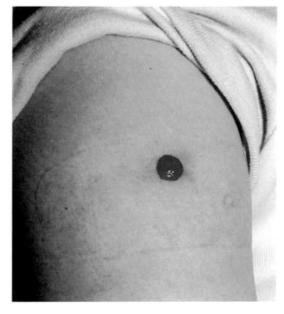

Figure 12.18 Pyogenic granuloma DLP ID: *pyogenic granuloma 2823*

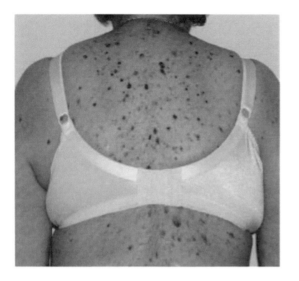

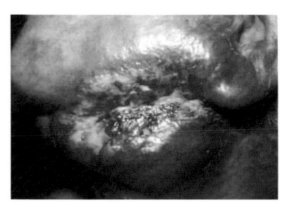

Figure 12.21 Syringoma, chondroid (mixed tumor of the skin). DLP ID: *syringoma, chondroid 933*

Figure 12.19 Seborrheic keratoses. DLP ID: *seborrheic keratoses 753*

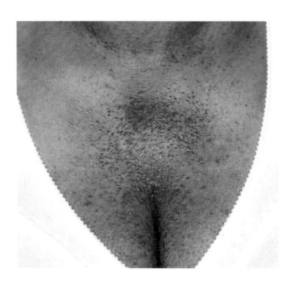

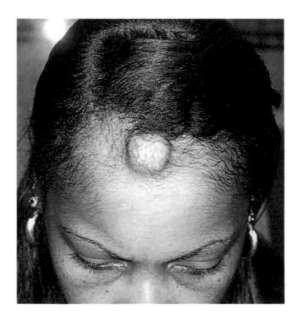

Figure 12.20 Steatocytoma multiplex. DLP ID: *steatocytoma multiplex 2885*

Figure 12.22 Tricholemmoma. DLP ID: *trichilemmoma 883*

MALIGNANT

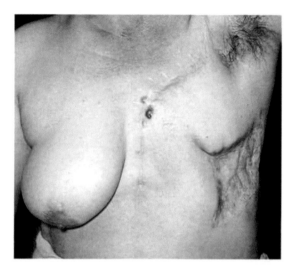

Figure 12.23 Adenocarcinoma of the breast, metastatic, post-mastectomy. DLP ID: *metastatic breast adenocarcinoma 1676*

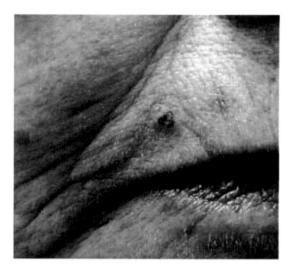

Figure 12.25 Basal cell carcinoma. DLP ID: *basal cell carcinoma 797*. Courtesy of Dr T Cestari, Porto Alegre, Brazil

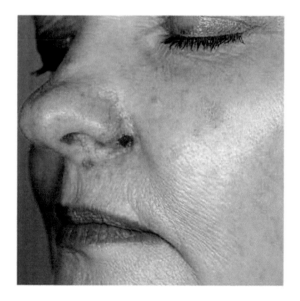

Figure 12.24 Basal cell carcinoma. DLP ID: *basal cell carcinoma 797*

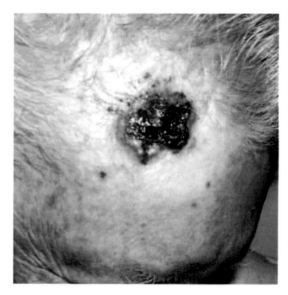

Figure 12.26 Basal cell carcinoma (rodent ulcer). DLP ID: *rodent ulcer of basal cell carcinoma 5222*. Courtesy of Dr T Cestari, Porto Alegre, Brazil

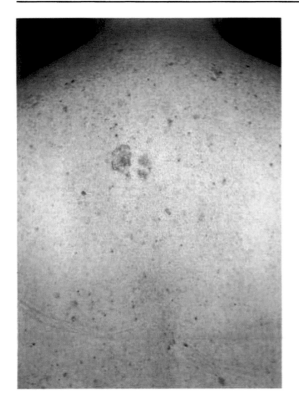

Figure 12.27 Basal cell nevus syndrome. DLP ID: *basal cell nevus syndrome 2883*

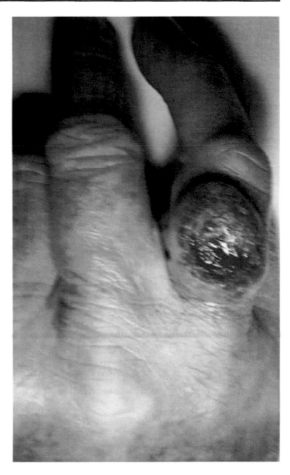

Figure 12.29 Keratoacanthoma. DLP ID: *keratoacanthoma 747*

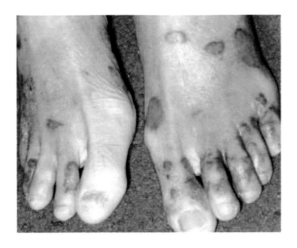

Figure 12.28 Kaposi's sarcoma in an immuno-competent patient. DLP ID: *Kaposi sarcoma 1457.* Courtesy of Drs L Guedes and G Munhoz-da-Fontoura, Rio de Janeiro, Brazil

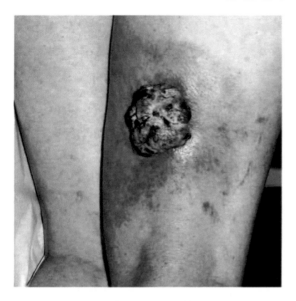

Figure 12.30 Melanoma, amelanotic. DLP ID: *melanoma, amelanotic 1068*

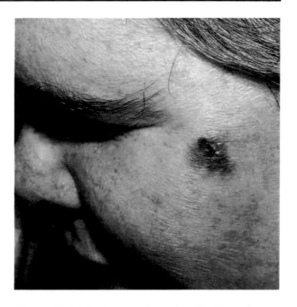

Figure 12.32 Melanoma, level 2. DLP ID: *malignant melanoma 4758*

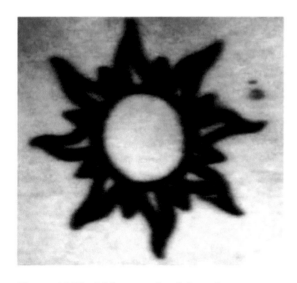

Figure 12.31 Melanoma, level 1 within a tattoo. DLP ID: *malignant melanoma 4758*

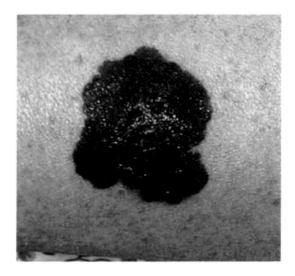

Figure 12.33 Melanoma, level 4. DLP ID: *malignant melanoma 4758*

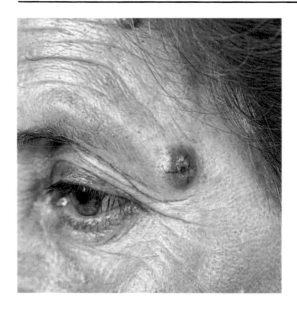

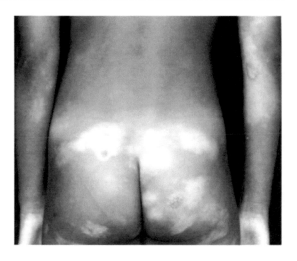

Figure 12.34 Merkel cell carcinoma. DLP ID: *Merkel cell carcinoma 1137*

Figure 12.36 Mycosis fungoides, hypopigmented (cutaneous T cell lymphoma). DLP ID: *hypopigmented mycosis fungoides 2813*. Courtesy of Dr S Carneiro, Rio de Janeiro, Brazil

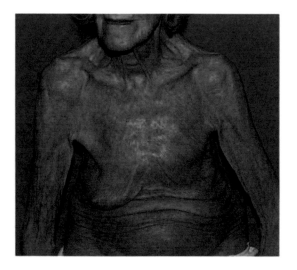

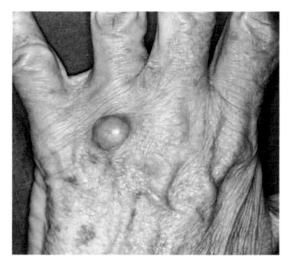

Figure 12.35 Mycosis fungoides, erythrodermic (cutaneous T cell lymphoma). DLP ID: *erythrodermic mycosis fungoides 1544*

Figure 12.37 Squamous cell carcinoma. DLP ID: *squamous cell carcinoma 798*

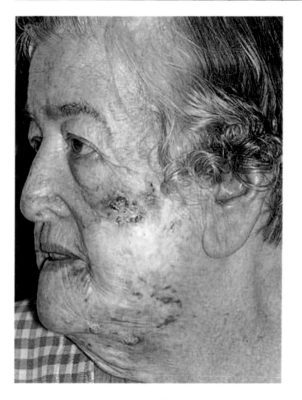

Figure 12.38 Squamous cell carcinoma. DLP ID: *squamous cell carcinoma 798*

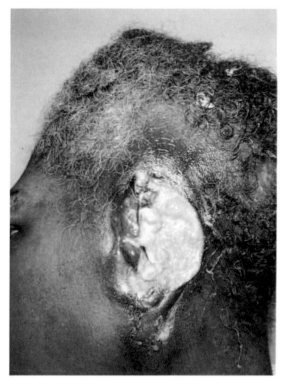

Figure 12.39 Squamous cell carcinoma. DLP ID: *squamous cell carcinoma 798*

Cutaneous manifestations of systemic diseases

13

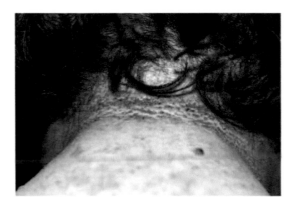

Figure 13.1 Acanthosis nigricans. Dermatology Lexicon Project (DLP) preferred term and number: *acanthosis nigricans 2797*

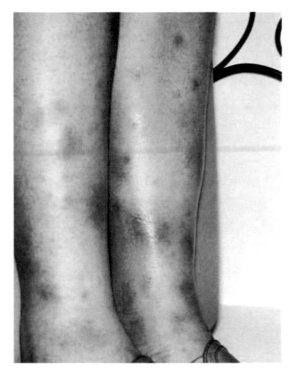

Figure 13.2 Erythema nodosum. DLP ID: *erythema nodosum 2353*

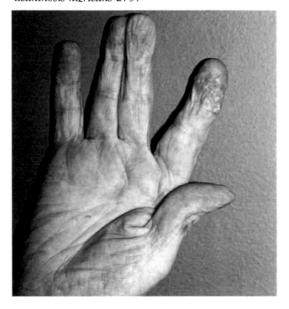

Figure 13.3 Gout. DLP ID: *gout 2594*

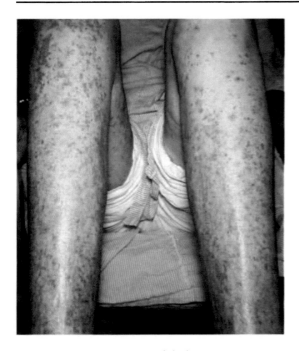

Figure 13.4 Hypergammaglobulinemia. DLP ID: *Waldenstrom macroglobulinemia 1802*

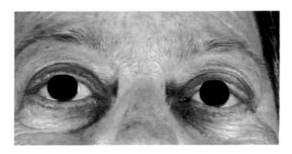

Figure 13.6 Hypothyroidism. DLP ID: *hypothyroidsm 1843*

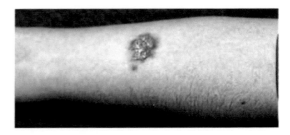

Figure 13.7 Necrobiois lipoidica diabeticorum. DLP ID: *necrobiois lipoidica diabeticorum 2197*

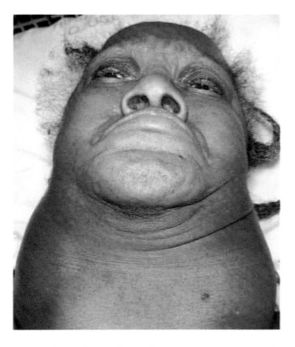

Figure 13.5 Hyperthyroidism – goiter. DLP ID: *hyperthyroidism goiter 1842*

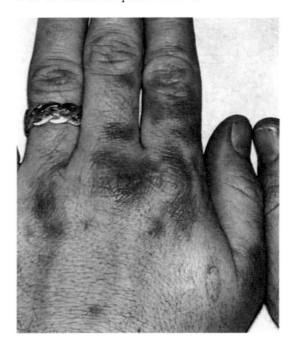

Figure 13.8 Porphyria cutanea tarda. DLP ID: *porphyria cutanea tarda 2575*

69

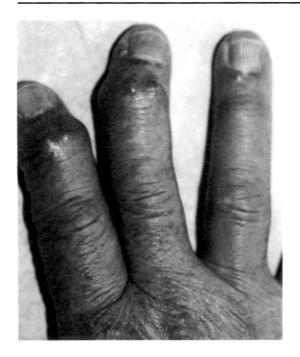

Figure 13.9 Reticulohistiocytosis, multicentric. DLP ID: *reticulohistiocytosis, multicentric 4383*

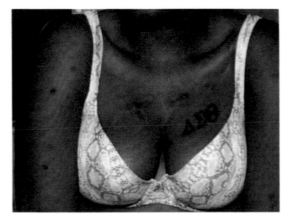

Figure 13.11 Sarcoidosis. DLP ID: *sarcoidosis 2203*

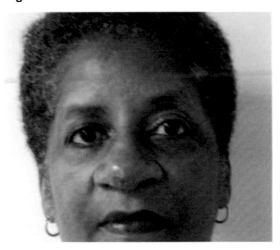

Figure 13.12 Sarcoidosis. DLP ID: *sarcoidosis 2203*

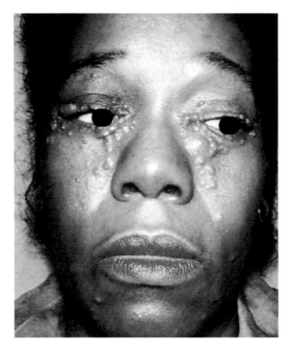

Figure 13.10 Sarcoidosis. DLP ID: *sarcoidosis 2203*

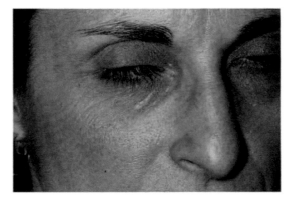

Figure 13.13 Xanthelasma. DLP ID: *xanthelasma 1610*

Drug eruptions

14

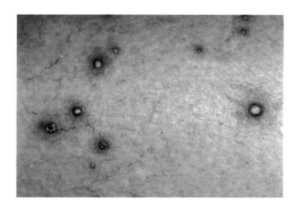

Figure 14.1 Acute generalized exanthematous pustulosis (AGEP) due to acetaminophen (paracetamol). Dermatology Lexicon Project (DLP) preferred term and number: *acute generalized exanthematous pustulosis 1894*

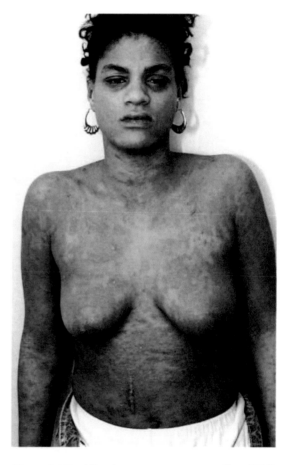

Figure 14.3 Allergic reaction to ampicillin. DLP ID: *exanthematous drug eruption 1889*

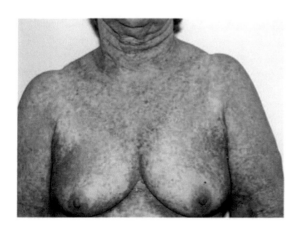

Figure 14.2 Allergic reaction to acetylsalicylic acid. DLP ID: *exanthematous drug eruption 1889*

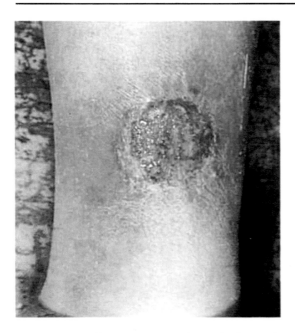

Figure 14.4 Allergic reaction to bromide (bromoderma) (originally included in Bromo-Seltzer®). DLP ID: *exanthematous drug eruption 1889*

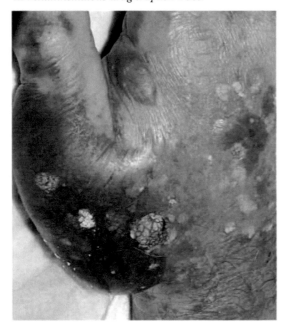

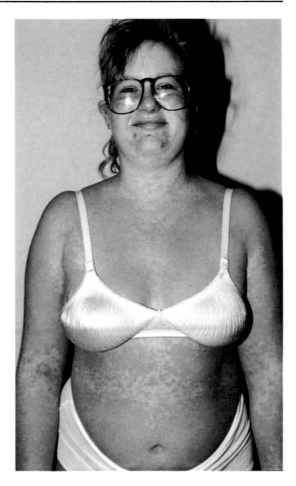

Figure 14.6 Allergic reaction to sulfonamide. DLP ID: *exanthematous drug eruption 1889*

Figure 14.5 Allergic reaction to penicillin (bullous eruption from an intravenous infusion). DLP ID: *exanthematous drug eruption 1889*

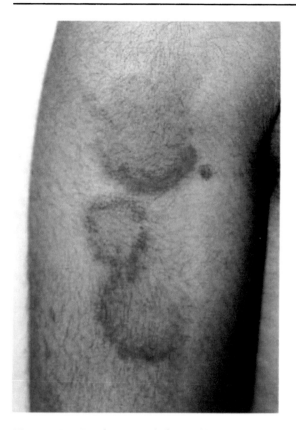

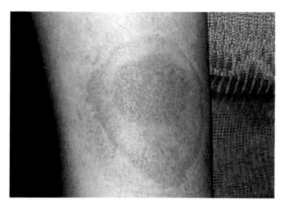

Figure 14.9 Fixed drug eruption due to tetracycline, pulsating (PFDE). DLP ID: *fixed drug eruption 1887*

Figure 14.7 Erythema multiforme-like drug eruption to acetylsalicylic acid. DLP ID: *erythema multiforme minor 4189*

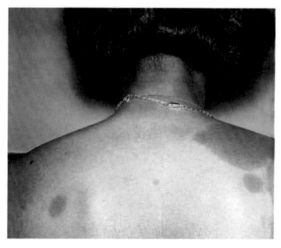

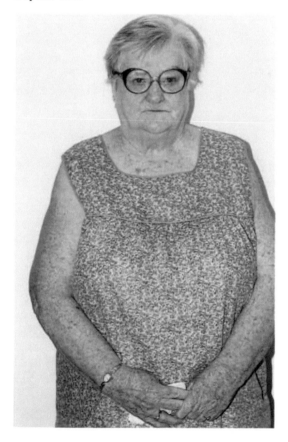

Figure 14.8 Fixed drug eruption due to phenolphthalein (FDE). DLP ID: *fixed drug eruption 1887*

Figure 14.10 Phototoxic drug eruption due to hydrochlorothiazide. DLP ID: *phototoxic reaction, drug induced 4181*

73

Psychodermatology

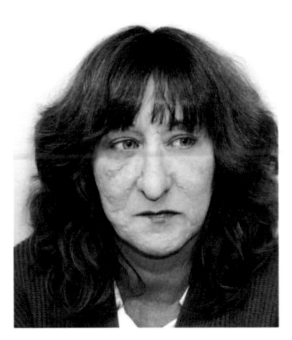

15

Figure 15.1 Acne excoriée and factitial dermatitis. Dermatology Lexicon Project (DLP) preferred term and number: *acne excoriee 653*

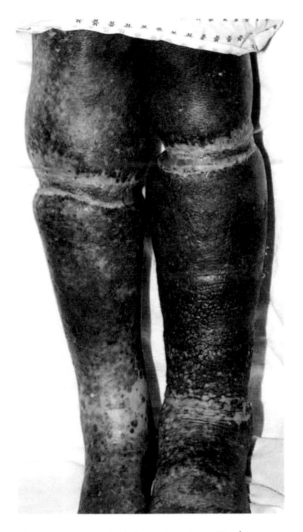

Figure 15.2 Factitial dermatitis. DLP ID: *dermatitis artefacta 617*

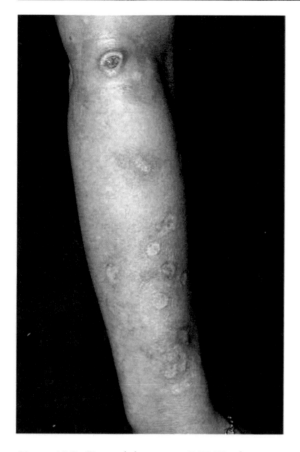

Figure 15.3 Factitial dermatitis. DLP ID: *dermatitis artefacta 617*

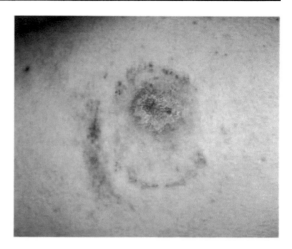

Figure 15.5 Human bite due to spousal abuse. DLP ID: *adult physical abuse 3875*

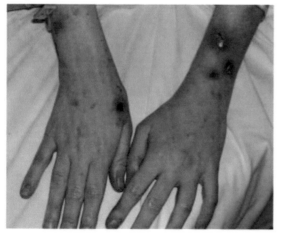

Figure 15.4 Factitial dermatitis. DLP ID: *dermatitis artefacta 617*

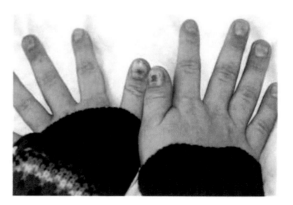

Figure 15.6 Nail dystrophy, median (picker's nail). DLP ID: *median nail dystrophy 4801*

75

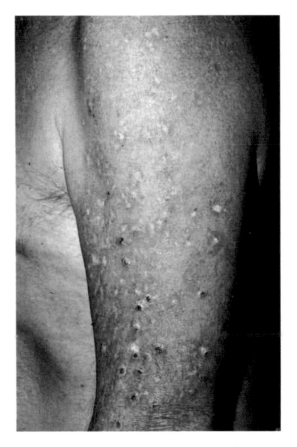

Figure 15.7 Neurotic excoriations. DLP ID: *dermatitis artefacta 617*

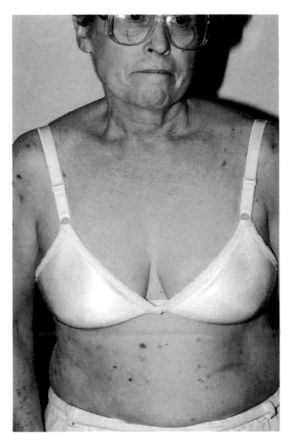

Figure 15.9 Parasitophobia. DLP ID: *delusion of parasitosis 689*

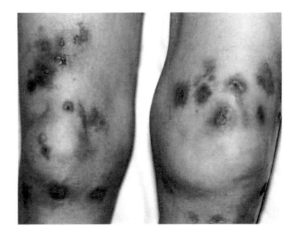

Figure 15.8 Neurotic excoriations. DLP ID: *dermatitis artefacta 617*

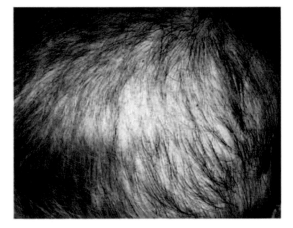

Figure 15.10 Trichotillomania. DLP ID: *trichotillomania 656*

Infections and infestations

Bacterial and mycobacterial diseases 16

BACTERIAL

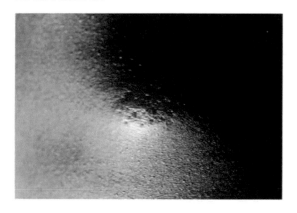

Figure 16.1 Anthrax (malignant pustule). Dermatology Lexicon Project (DLP) preferred term and number: *cutaneous anthrax 109*. Courtesy of Dr W Höffler, Tübingen, Germany

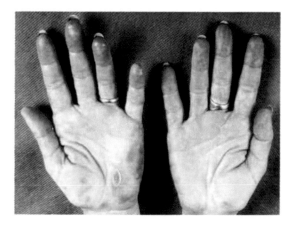

Figure 16.3 Cat scratch disease. DLP ID: *cat scratch disease 124*

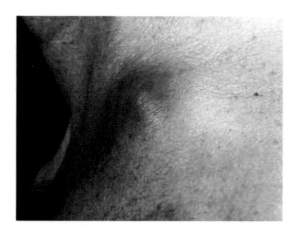

Figure 16.2 Cat scratch disease. DLP ID: *cat scratch disease 124*

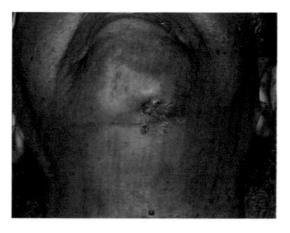

Figure 16.4 Dental sinus. DLP ID: *dental sinus 148*

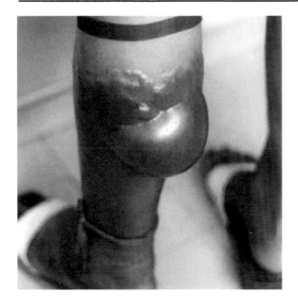

Figure 16.5 Erysipelas, bullous. DLP ID: *erysipelas 56*

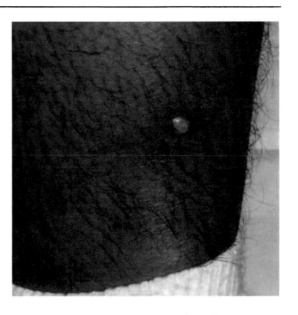

Figure 16.7 Furuncle. DLP ID: *furuncle 24*

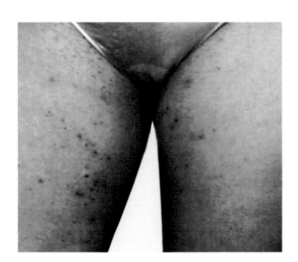

Figure 16.6 Folliculitis due to waxing. DLP ID: *folliculitis 23*

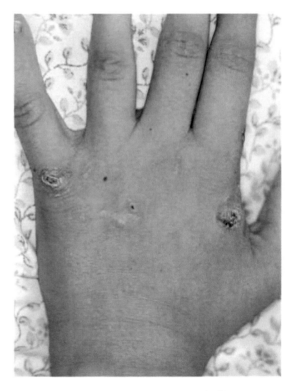

Figure 16.8 Impetigo. DLP ID: *non-bullous impetigo 19*

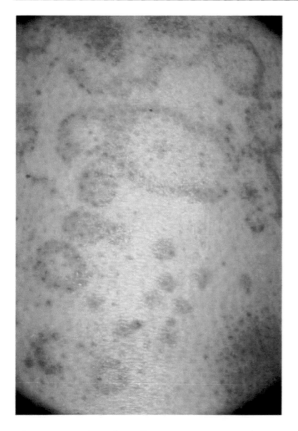

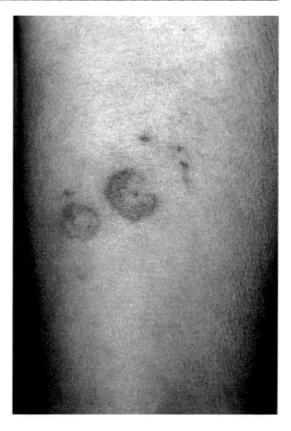

Figure 16.9 Lyme borreliosis. DLP ID: *Lyme disease 255*

Figure 16.10 Lyme borreliosis. DLP ID: *Lyme disease 255*

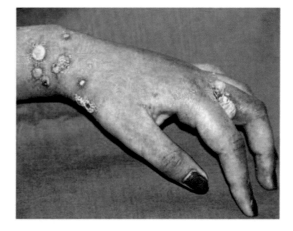

Figure 16.11 Pyoderma secondary to scabies. DLP ID: *scabies infestation 463*

MYCOBACTERIAL

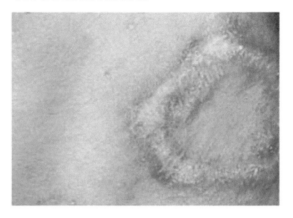

Figure 16.13 Leprosy, borderline. DLP ID: *border-line leprosy 182*. Courtesy of Dr JHS Pettit, Kuala Lumpur, Malaysia

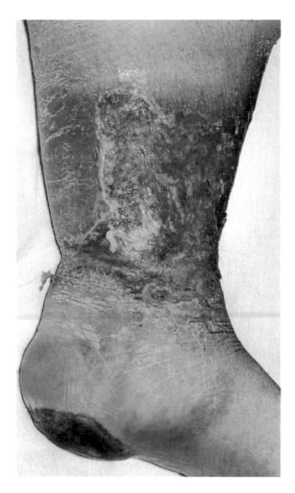

Figure 16.12 Pyoderma secondary to stasis ulcer. DLP ID: *statis ulcer 2514*

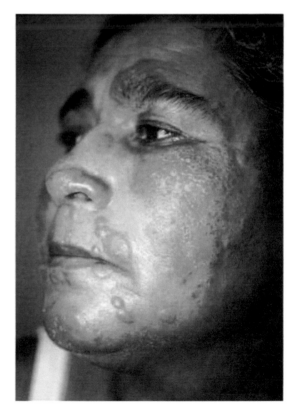

Figure 16.14 Leprosy, lepromatous. DLP ID: *borderline lepromatous leprosy 183*

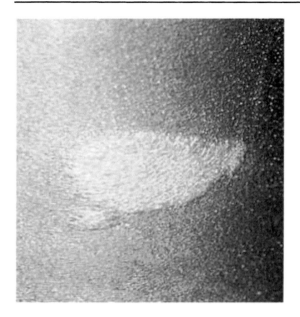

Figure 16.15 Leprosy, tuberculoid. DLP ID: *border-line tuberculoid leprosy 181*. Courtesy of Dr B Flageul, Paris, France

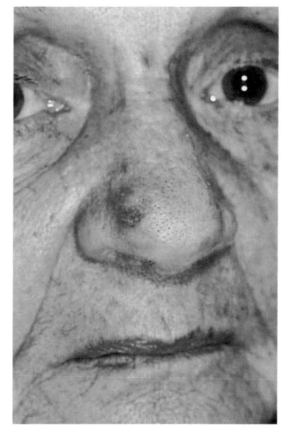

Figure 16.17 Lupus vulgaris. DLP ID: *lupus vulgaris 166*

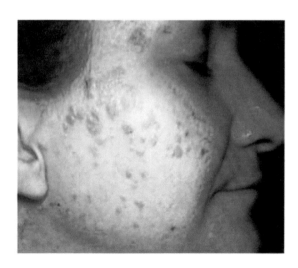

Figure 16.16 Lupus miliaris disseminatus faciei. DLP ID: *granulomatous rosacea 2312*

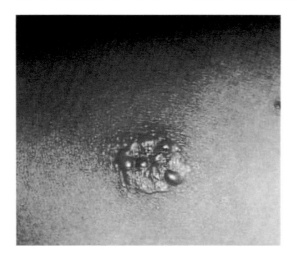

Figure 16.18 Papulonecrotic tuberculid. DLP ID: *papulonecrotic tuberculid 172*

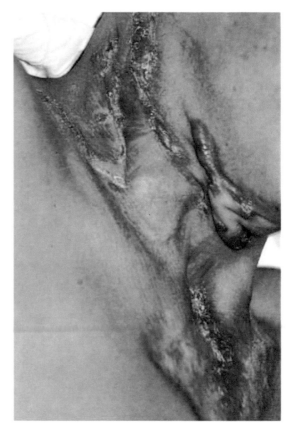

Figure 16.19 Scrofuloderma. DLP ID: *scrofulo-derma 167.* Courtesy of Dr KD Pramatarov, Sofia, Bulgaria

Rickettsial diseases

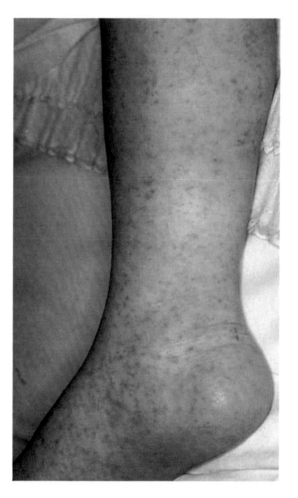

Figure 17.1 Rocky Mountain spotted fever. Dermatology Lexicon Project (DLP) preferred term and number: *Rocky Mountain spotted fever 227*

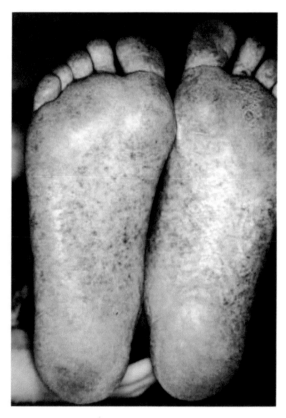

Figure 17.2 Typhus due to *Rickettsia conorii*. DLP ID: *boutonneuse fever 236*

Viral diseases 18

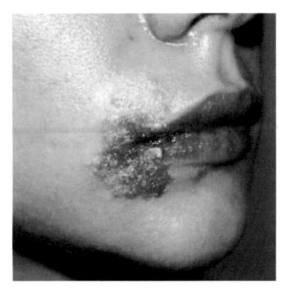

Figure 18.1 Herpes simplex labialis. Dermatology Lexicon Project (DLP) preferred term and number: *orolabial herpes simplex 501. Courtesy of Dr I Botev, Sofia, Bulgaria*

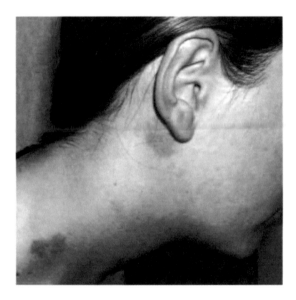

Figure 18.2 Herpes zoster. DLP ID: *herpes zoster virus infection 497*

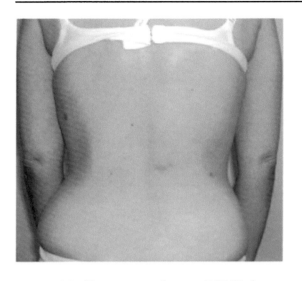

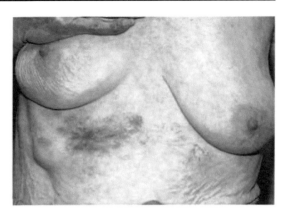

Figure 18.5 Herpes zoster with keloid formation. DLP ID: *herpes zoster virus infection 497 combined wih keloid 1264*

Figure 18.3 Herpes zoster, day one. DLP ID: *herpes zoster virus infection 497*

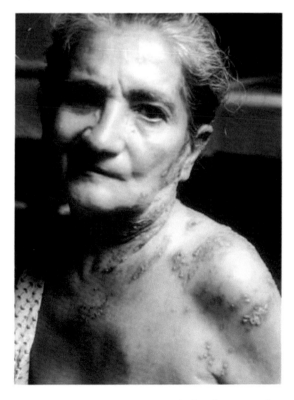

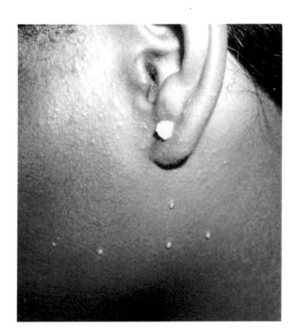

Figure 18.4 Herpes zoster with facial nerve palsy (Ramsay Hunt syndrome). DLP ID: *herpes zoster virus infection 497*

Figure 18.6 Molluscum contagiosum. DLP ID: *molluscum contagiosum 575*

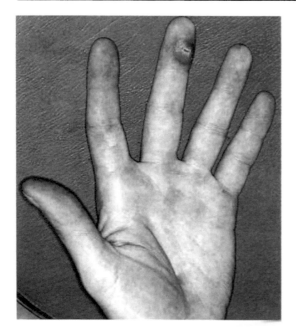

Figure 18.7 Orf (ecthyma contagiosum). DLP ID: *orf 580*

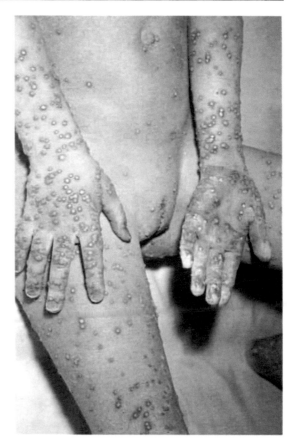

Figure 18.9 Variola (smallpox). DLP ID: *smallpox 576*. Courtesy of Dr G Stüttgen, Berlin, Germany

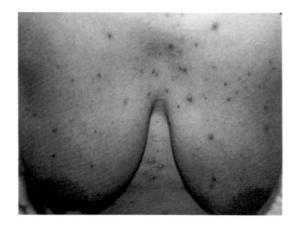

Figure 18.8 Varicella (chickenpox). DLP ID: *varicella virus infection 496*

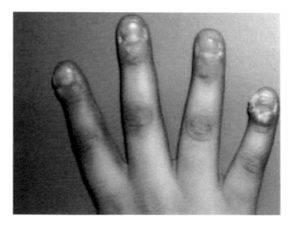

Figure 18.10 Verrucae. DLP ID: *verruca vulgaris 598*

Superficial and deep fungal diseases 19

SUPERFICIAL FUNGAL DISEASES

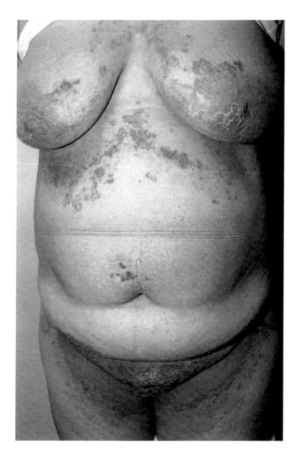

Figure 19.1 Candidosis. Dermatology Lexicon Project (DLP) preferred term and number: *candidiasis 296*

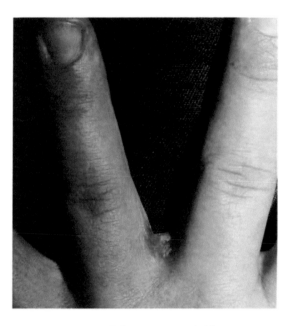

Figure 19.2 Candidosis (pseudoblastomycosis interdigitale). DLP ID: *erosio interdigitalis blastomycetica candidiasis 360*

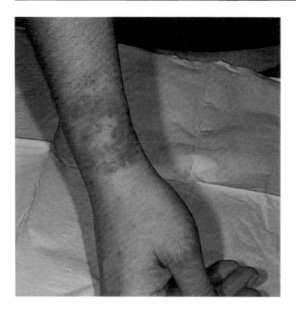

Figure 19.3 Majocchi's granuloma. DLP ID; *Majocchi granuloma 338*

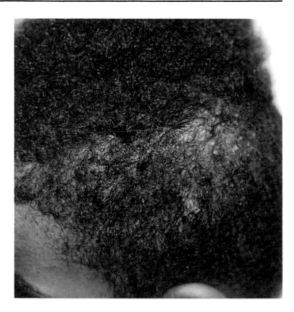

Figure 19.5 Tinea capitis with kerion formation. DLP ID: *tinea capitis 321 combined with kerion 334*

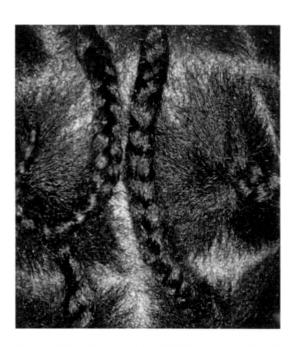

Figure 19.4 Tinea capitis. DLP ID: *tinea capitis 321*

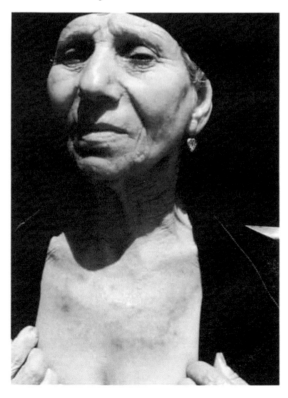

Figure 19.6 Tinea corporis. DLP ID: *tinea corporis 324*

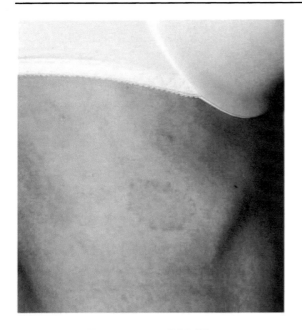

Figure 19.7 Tinea corporis. DLP ID: *tinea corporis 324*

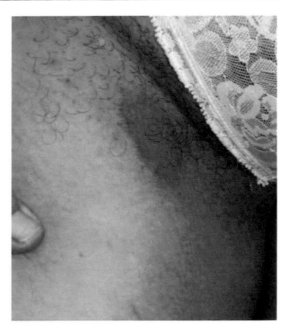

Figure 19.9 Tinea cruris. DLP ID: *tinea cruris 327*. Courtesy of Dr N Fernandes, Rio de Janeiro, Brazil

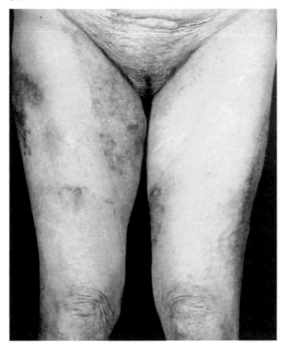

Figure 19.8 Tinea corporis augmented by topical steroids (tinea incognito). DLP ID: *tinea incognito 326*

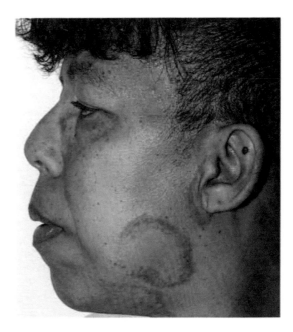

Figure 19.10 Tinea faciei. DLP ID: *tinea faciale 325*

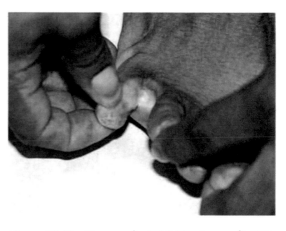

Figure 19.13   Tinea pedis. DLP ID: *tinea pedis 328*

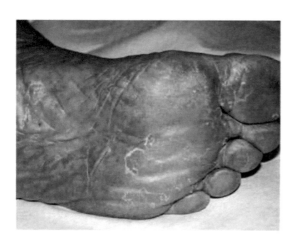

Figure 19.11   Tinea nigra. DLP ID: *tinea nigra 342.*
Courtesy of Dr N Fernandes, Rio de Janeiro, Brazil

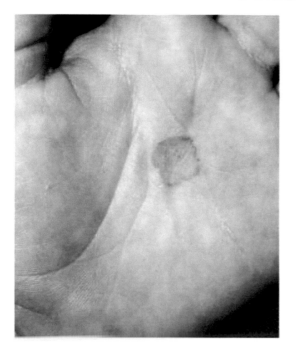

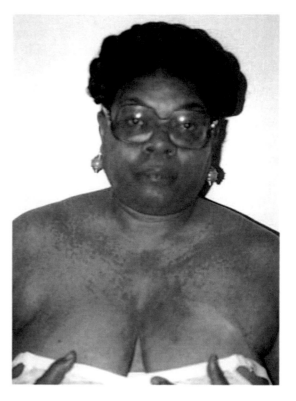

Figure 19.12   Tinea pedis. DLP ID: *tinea pedis 328*

Figure 19.14   Tinea versicolor. DLP ID: *tinea versicolor 343*

SUBCUTANEOUS AND DEEP FUNGAL DISEASES

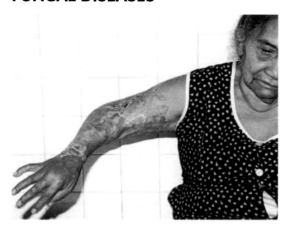

Figure 19.15 Chromoblastomycosis. DLP ID: *chromoblastomycosis 299*

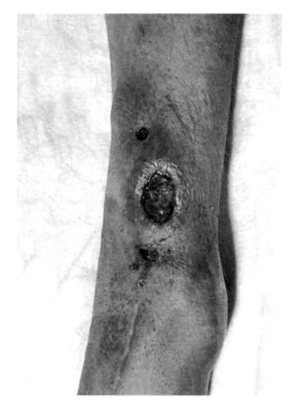

Figure 19.17 Cryptococcosis. DLP ID: *cryptococcosis 309*. Courtesy of Dr S Sampaio, Sao Paulo, Brazil

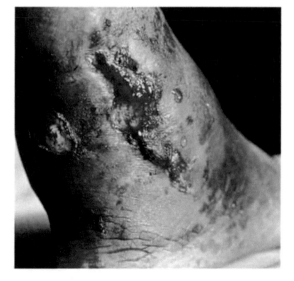

Figure 19.16 Coccidiomycosis. DLP ID: *coccidioidomycosis 310*. Courtesy of Dr JHS Pettit, Kuala Lumpur, Malaysia

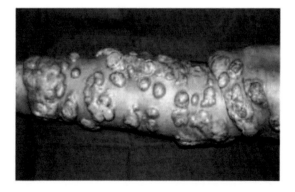

Figure 19.18 Lobomycosis. DLP ID: *lobomycosis 302*. Courtesy of Dr A de Brito, Rio de Janeiro, Brazil

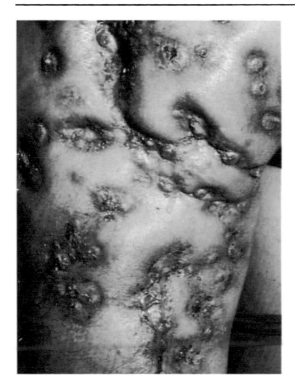

Figure 19.19 Mycetoma. DLP ID: *mycetoma 388*

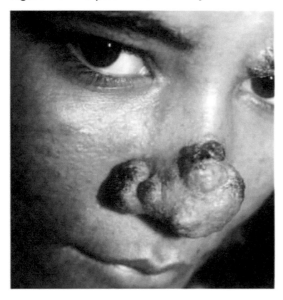

Figure 19.20 Paracoccidioidomycosis   (South American   blastomycosis).   DLP   ID: *paracoccidioidomycosis 308*

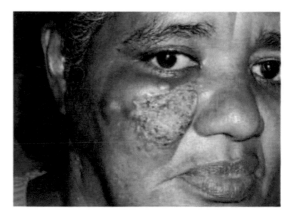

Figure 19.21 Sporotrichosis. DLP ID: *sporotrichosis 298*. Courtesy of Drs N Fernandes and G Munhoz-da-Fontoura, Rio de Janeiro, Brazil

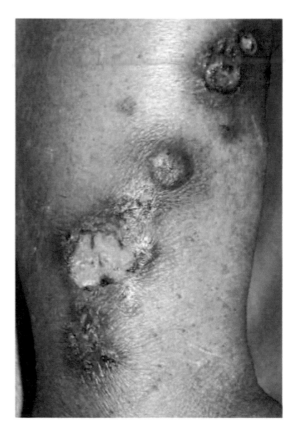

Figure 19.22 Sporotrichosis in a woman with multiple myeloma. DLP ID: *sporotrichosis 298*

Parasitic diseases

20

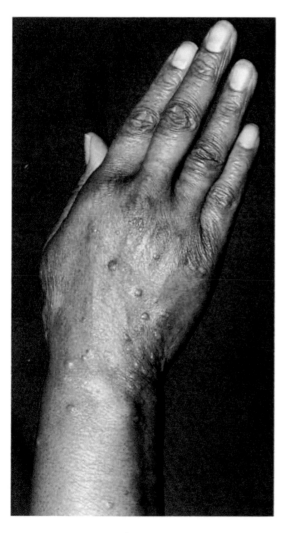

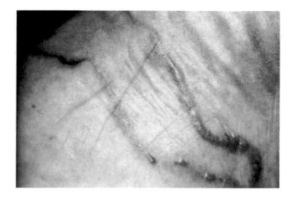

Figure 20.2 Larva migrans. DLP ID: *cutaneous larva migrans 417*. Courtesy of Dr W Höffler, Tübingen, Germany

Figure 20.1 Insect bite reaction. Dermatology Lexicon Project (DLP) preferred term and number: *arthropod bite 3596*

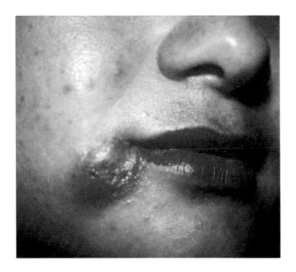

Figure 20.3 Leishmaniasis, cutaneous American. DLP ID: *New World leishmaniasis 407*

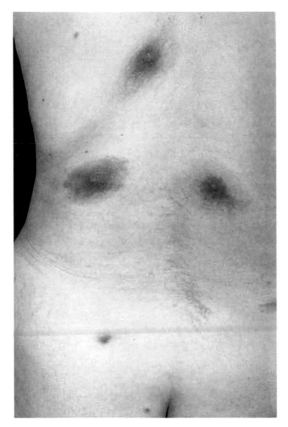

Figure 20.5 Myiasis. DLP ID: myiasis *464*

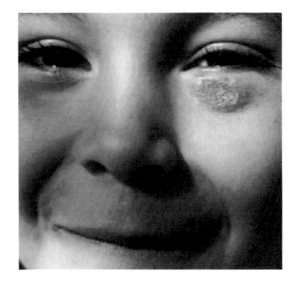

Figure 20.4 Leishmaniasis, cutaneous American. DLP ID: *New World leishmaniasis 407*

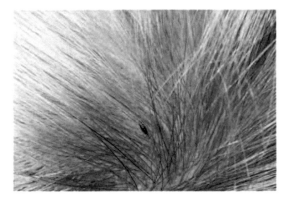

Figure 20.6 Pediculosis capitis. DLP ID: *pediculosis capitis 465*

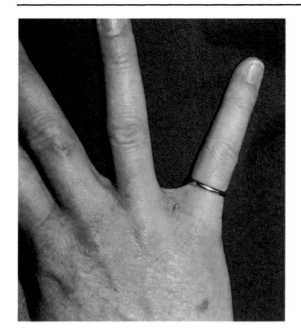

Figure 20.7 Scabies. DLP ID: *scabies infestation 463*

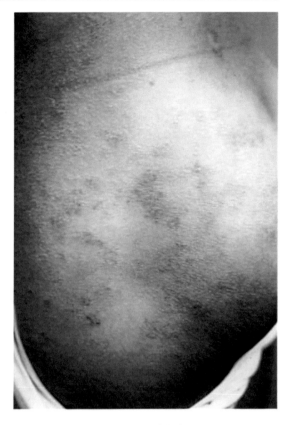

Figure 20.9 Scabies in an elderly patient. DLP ID: *scabies infestation 463*

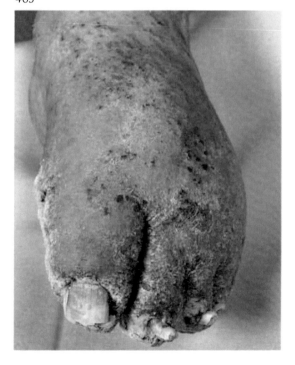

Figure 20.8 Scabies, crusted. DLP ID: *crusted scabies 469*

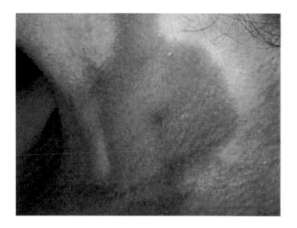

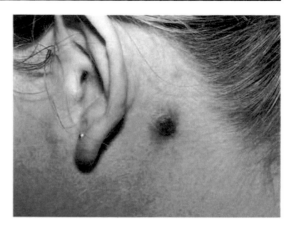

Figure 20.10 Spider bite, type unknown. DLP ID: *spider bite 3642*

Figure 20.11 Tick bite. DLP ID: *tick bite 3654*

Sexually transmitted disease and AIDS 21

SEXUALLY TRANSMITTED DISEASES

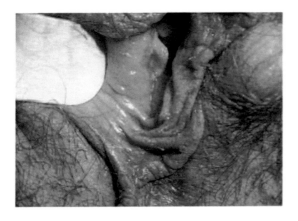

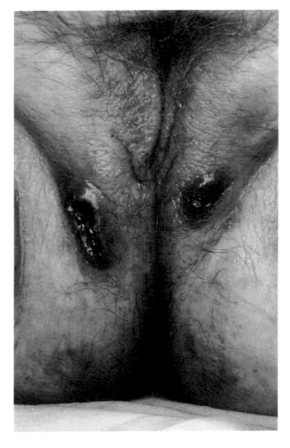

Figure 21.2 Granuloma inguinale. DLP ID: *granuloma inguinale 88*. Courtesy of Dr B Fisher, Tel Aviv, Israel

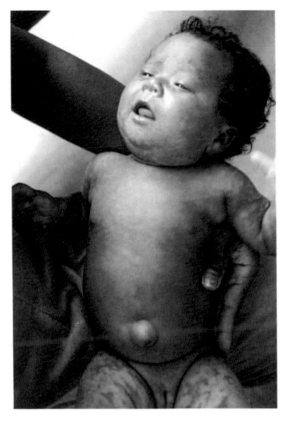

Figure 21.3 Syphilis, congenital. DLP ID: *congenital syphilis 271*

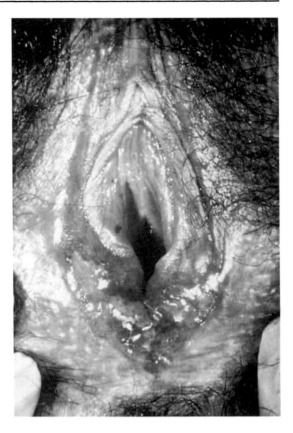

Figure 21.4 Syphilis, primary. DLP ID: *primary syphilis 268*

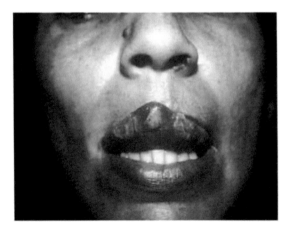

Figure 21.5 Syphilis, secondary. DLP ID: *secondary syphilis 269*

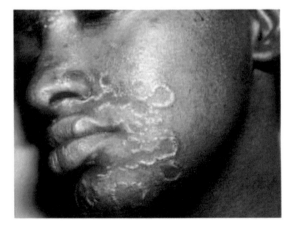

Figure 21.6 Syphilis, secondary. DLP ID: *secondary syphilis 269*

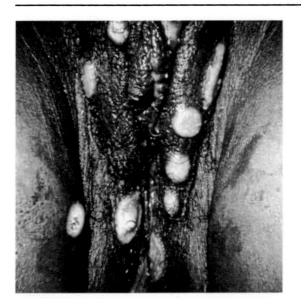

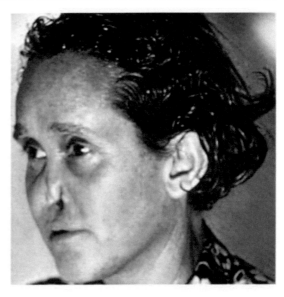

Figure 21.7 Syphilis, secondary – condylomata lata. DLP ID: *condyloma lata of secondary syphilis 273*

Figure 21.8 Syphilis tertiary. DLP ID: *tertiary syphilis 270*

AIDS

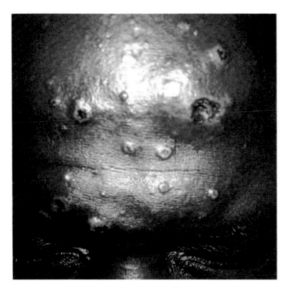

Figure 21.9 Cryptococcosis in an AIDS patient. DLP ID: *cryptococcosis 309*. Courtesy of Drs NC Dlova and A Mosam, Durban, South Africa

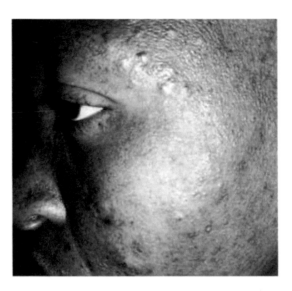

Figure 21.11 Eosinophilic folliculitis in an AIDS patient. DLP ID: *eosinophilic folliculitis 2323*. Courtesy of Drs NC Dlova and A Mosam, Durban, South Africa

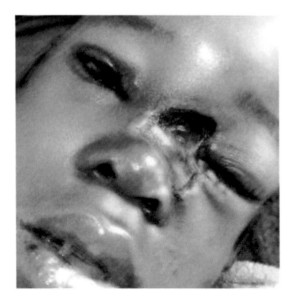

Figure 21.10 Cytomegalovirus infection (CMV) in an AIDS patient. DLP ID: *cytomegalovirus infection 499*. Courtesy of Drs NC Dlova and A Mosam, Durban, South Africa

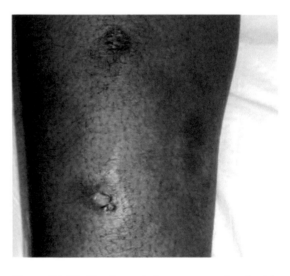

Figure 21.12 Erythema induratum associated with tuberculosis in an AIDS patient. DLP ID: *erythema induratum 2356*. Courtesy of Drs NC Dlova and A Mosam, Durban, South Africa

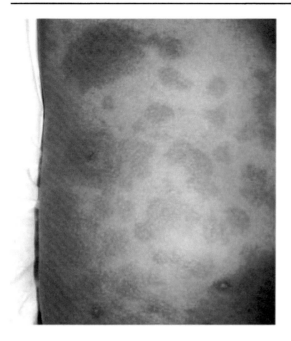

Figure 21.13 Erythema multiforme due to trimethoprim-sulfamethoxazole in an AIDS patient. DLP ID: *erythema multiforme major 1876*. Courtesy of Drs NC Dlova and A Mosam, Durban, South Africa

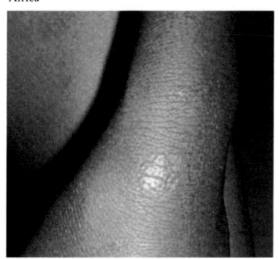

Figure 20.14 Fixed drug eruption (DE) due to trimethoprim-sulfamethoxazole in an AIDS patient. DLP ID: *fixed drug eruption 1887*. Courtesy of Drs NC Dlova and A Mosam, Durban, South Africa

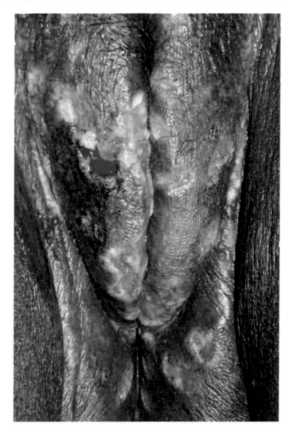

Figure 21.15 Herpes progenitalis in an AIDS patient. DLP ID: *genital herpes simplex 502*. Courtesy of Drs NC Dlova and A Mosam, Durban, South Africa

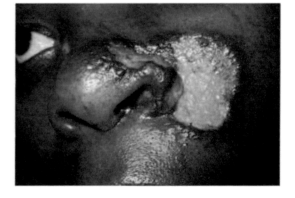

Figure 21.16 Histoplasmosis in an AIDS patient. DLP ID: *histoplasmosis 306*. Courtesy of Drs NC Dlova and A Mosam, Durban, South Africa

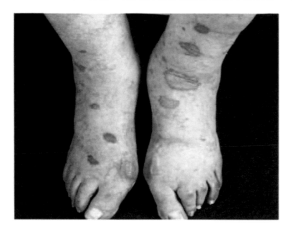

Figure 21.17 Kaposi's sarcoma in an AIDS patient. DLP ID: *immunosuppression-related Kaposi sarcoma 1457*

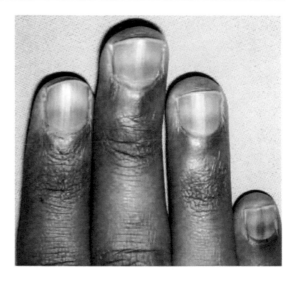

Figure 21.19 Melanonychia following zidovudine (AZT) therapy in an AIDS patient. DLP ID: *melanonychia striata 1082.* Courtesy of Drs NC Dlova and A Mosam, Durban, South Africa

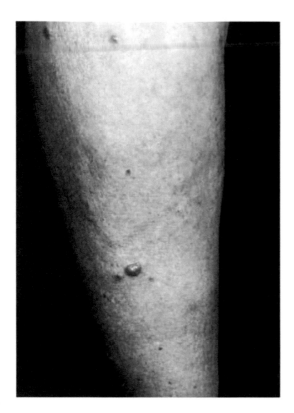

Figure 21.18 Kaposi's sarcoma in an AIDS patient. DLP ID: *immunosuppression-related Kaposi sarcoma 1457*

Topographic dermatology

Diseases of the breast

22

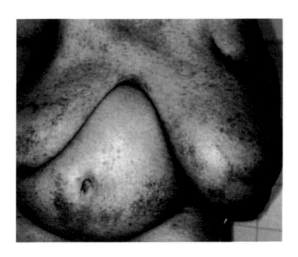

Figure 22.1 Abscess. Dermatology Lexicon Project (DLP) preferred term and number: *abscess 34*

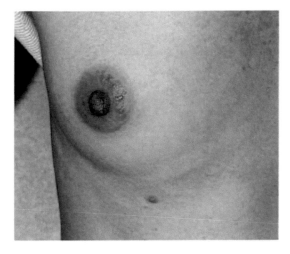

Figure 22.2 Accessory (supernumerary) nipple. DLP ID: *accessory nipple 4314*

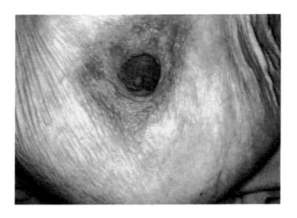

Figure 22.3 Adenomatosis, erosive. DLP ID: *nipple erosive adenomatosis 924*

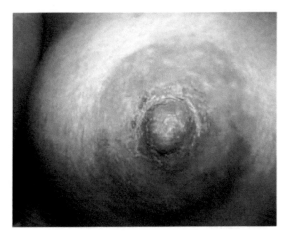

Figure 22.4 Atopic dermatitis. DLP ID: *atopic dermatitis 2100*

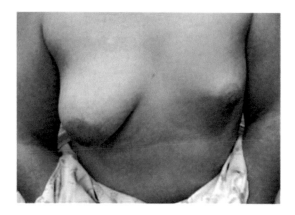

Figure 22.5 Breast, hypoplastic. DLP ID: *hypoplastic breast 6677*

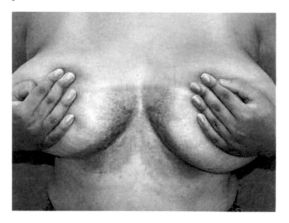

Figure 22.6 Candidosis. DLP ID: *candidiasis 296*

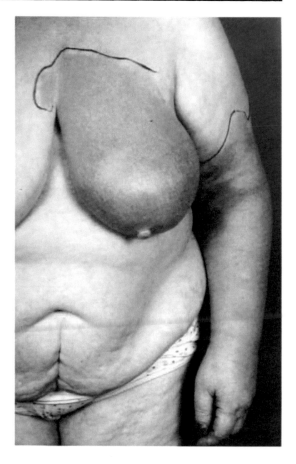

Figure 22.8 Erysipelas, post-lumpectomy 13 years prior. DLP ID: *erysipelas 56*

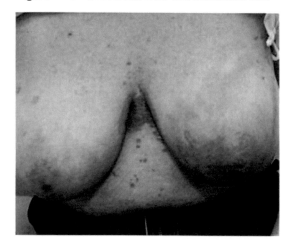

Figure 22.7 Candidosis. DLP ID: *candidiasis 296*

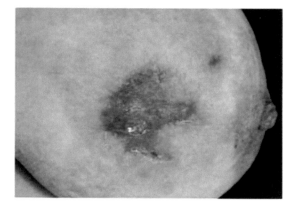

Figure 22.9 Factitial dermatitis. DLP ID: *dermatitis artefacta 617*

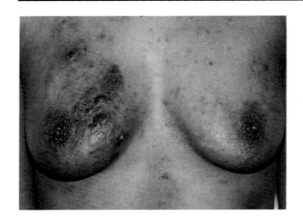

Figure 22.10 Keloids. DLP ID: *keloid 1264*

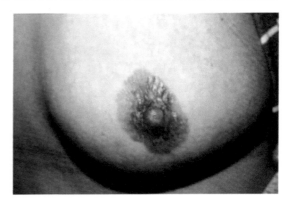

Figure 22.12 Paget's disease. DLP ID: *Paget disease of breast 4549*

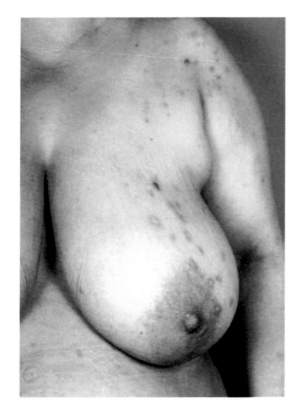

Figure 22.11 Neurotic excoriations. DLP ID: *dermatitis artefacta 617*

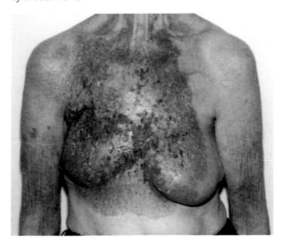

Figure 22.13 Paget's disease. DLP ID: *Paget disease of breast 4549*

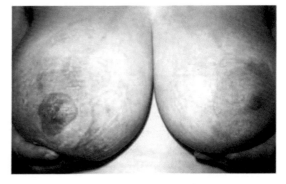

Figure 22.14 Paget's disease disc. DLP ID: *Paget disease of breast 4549*

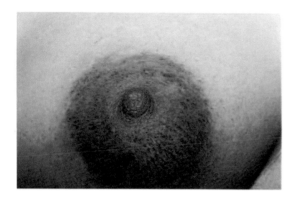

Figure 22.15 Seborrheic keratosis. DLP ID: *seborrheic keratosis 753*

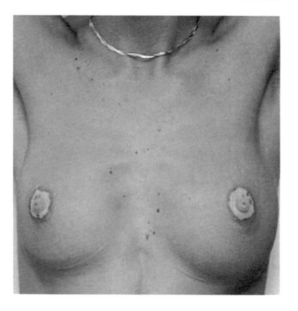

Figure 22.17 Vitiligo. DLP ID: *vitiligo 1839*

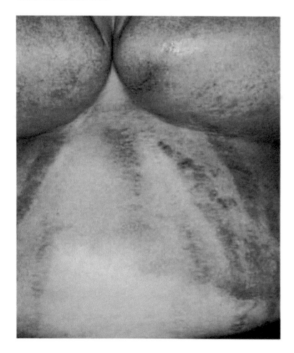

Figure 22.16 Striae due to chronic use of a potent steroid/antifungal cream. DLP ID: *striae due to topical corticosteroid 4212*

Oral lesions

23

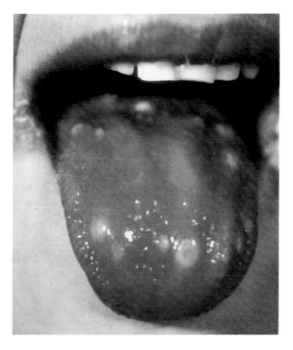

Figure 23.1 Aphthous stomatitis, etiology undetermined. Dermatology Lexicon Project (DLP) preferred term and number: *aphthous stomatitis 2331*

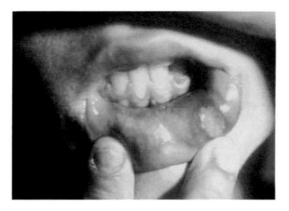

Figure 23.2 Behçet's disease. DLP ID: *Behçet's disease 2166*

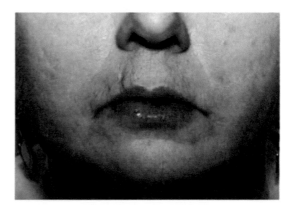

Figure 23.3 Cheilitis, actinic. DLP ID: *actinic cheilitis 776*

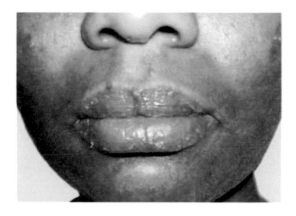

Figure 23.4 Cheilitis due to oral isotretinoin therapy. DLP ID: *cheilitis, drug induced 4227*

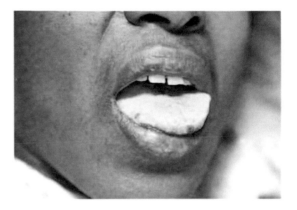

Figure 23.6 Herpes simplex labialis, primary infection. DLP ID: *orolabial herpes simplex 501*

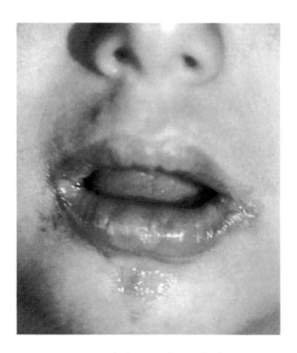

Figure 23.5 Hand, foot, and mouth disease. DLP ID: *hand-foot-mouth disease 565*

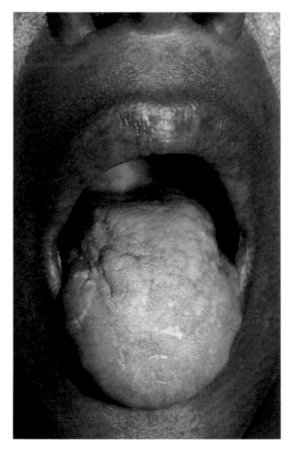

Figure 23.7 Lichen planus. DLP ID: *lichen planus 4843*

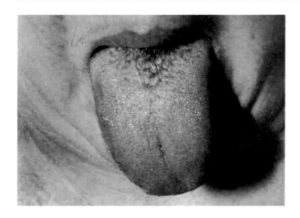

Figure 23.8 Lingua nigra. DLP ID: *black tongue 4235*

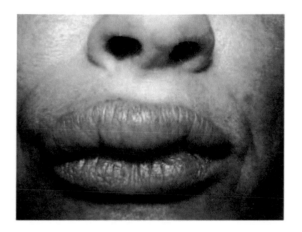

Figure 23.9 Melkersson-Rosenthal syndrome. DLP ID: *Melkersson-Rosenthal syndrome 705*

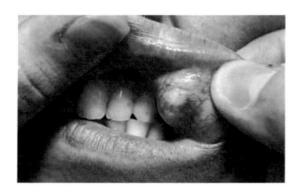

Figure 23.10 Mucocele. DLP ID: *mucocele 851*

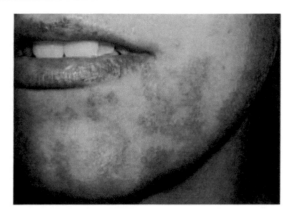

Figure 23.11 Osler-Weber-Rendu syndrome. DLP ID: *hereditary hemorrhagic telangiectasia 1411.* Courtesy of Drs C Sodre and G Munhoz-da-Fontoura, Rio de Janeiro, Brazil

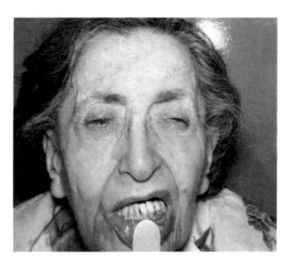

Figure 23.12 Pemphigoid, cicatricial. DLP ID: *cicatricial pemphigoid 1761*

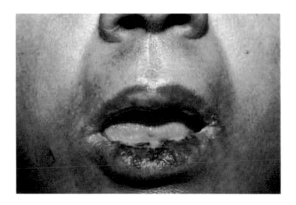

Figure 23.13 Pemphigus foliaceus. DLP ID: *pemphigus foliaceus 1750*

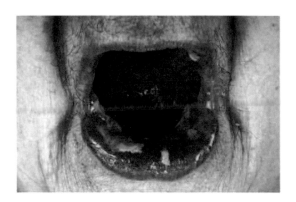

Figure 23.14 Pemphigus vulgaris. DLP ID: *pemphigus vulgaris 1748*

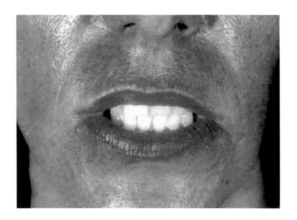

Figure 23.15 Peutz-Jeghers syndrome. DLP ID: *Peutz-Jeghers syndrome 3245*

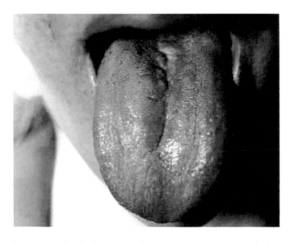

Figure 23.16 Pseudoepitheliomatous hyperplasia. DLP ID: *pseudopitheliomatous hyperplasia 738*. Courtesy of Dr O Oumeish, Amman, Jordan

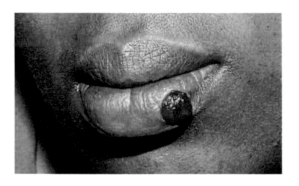

Figure 23.17 Pyogenic granuloma. DLP ID: *pyogenic granuloma 2823*

Perineal and perianal diseases 24

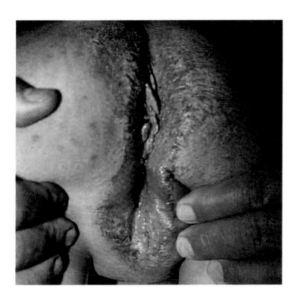

Figure 24.1 Candidosis, chronic mucocutaneous and condyloma acuminata. Dermatology Lexicon Project (DLP) preferred term and number: *chronic mucocutaneous candidiasis 364*

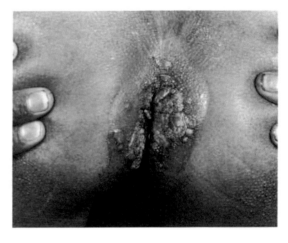

Figure 24.2 Condyloma acuminata. DLP ID: *condyloma acuminata 603*

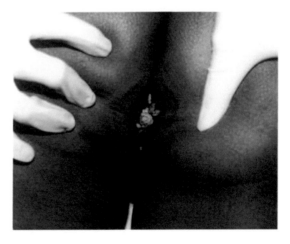

Figure 24.3 Condyloma acuminata. DLP ID: *condyloma acuminata 603*

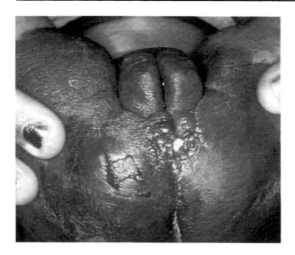

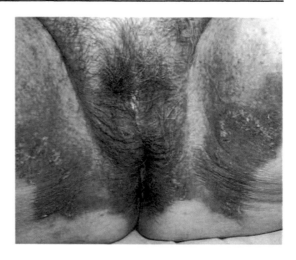

Figure 24.4 Nevus, congenital. DLP ID: *congenital nevus 1020*

Figure 24.6 Pemphigus, benign familial chronic (Hailey–Hailey disease). DLP ID: *Hailey–Hailey disease 3503*

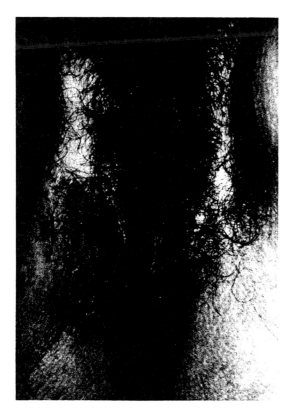

Figure 24.5 Paget's disease, extramammary. DLP ID: *Paget disease 966*

Diseases of the vulva

25

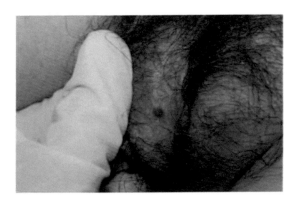

Figure 25.1 Angioma. Dermatology Lexicon Project (DLP) preferred term and number: *hemangioma, unclassified 5263*

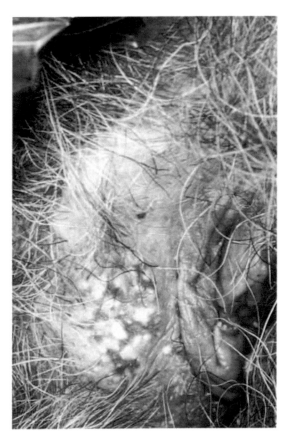

Figure 25.2 Basal cell carcinoma. DLP ID: *basal cell carcinoma 797*

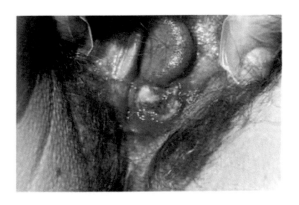

Figure 25.3 Behçet's disease. DLP ID: *Behçet's disease 2166*

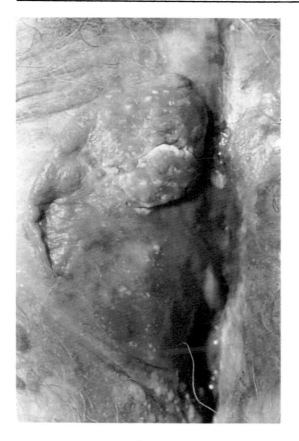

Figure 25.4 Bowen's disease (squamous cell carcinoma, intraepidermal). DLP ID: *squamous cell carcinoma in-situ 788*

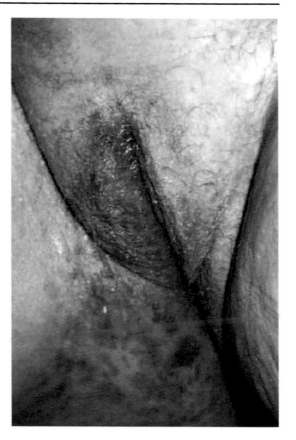

Figure 25.6 Herpes zoster. DLP ID: *herpes zoster virus infection 497*

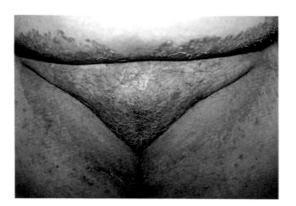

Figure 25.5 Candidosis. DLP ID: *candidiasis 296*

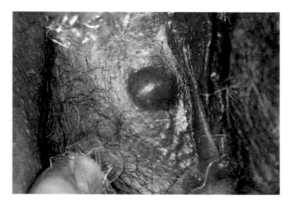

Figure 25.7 Hidradenoma papilliferum. DLP ID: *hidradenoma papilliferum 917*

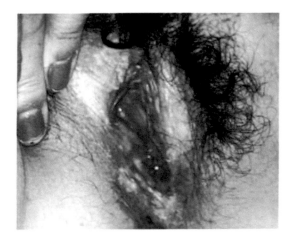

Figure 25.8 Lichen sclerosus et atrophicus. DLP ID: *lichen sclerosus 2263*

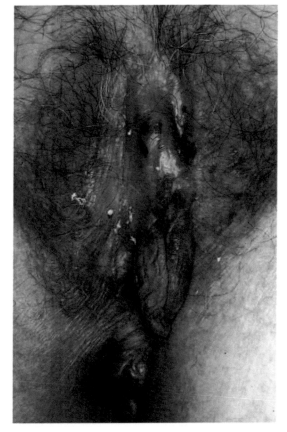

Figure 25.10 Melanoma. DLP ID: *malignant melanoma 4758*

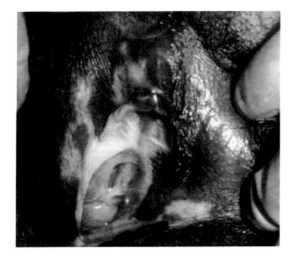

Figure 25.9 Lichen sclerosus et atrophicus. DLP ID: *lichen sclerosus 2263*

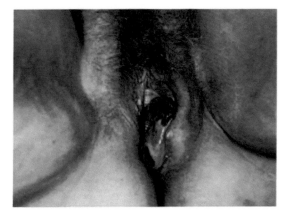

Figure 25.11 Melanoma, level V with metastasis. DLP ID: *malignant melanoma 4758*. Courtesy of Dr B Fisher, Tel Aviv, Israel

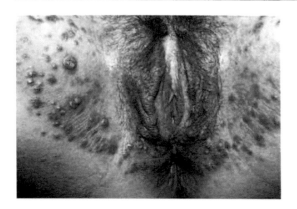

Figure 25.12 Molluscum contagiosum. DLP ID: *molluscum contagiosum 575*

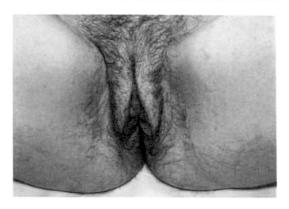

Figure 25.14 Pruritus vulva. DLP ID: *pruritus vulvae 648*

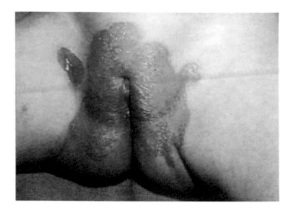

Figure 25.15 Psoriasis inversus. DLP ID: *inverse psoriasis 2083*. Courtesy of Dr B Fisher, Tel Aviv, Israel

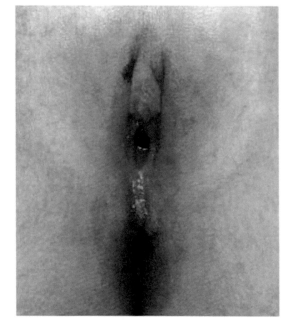

Figure 25.13 Nevus, junctional. DLP ID: *junctional nevus 1006*. Courtesy of Dr B Fisher, Tel Aviv, Israel

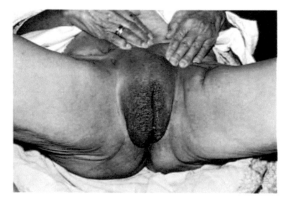

Figure 25.16 Scrofuloderma. DLP ID: *scrofuloderma 167*. Courtesy of Dr M Sollimon, Cairo, Egypt

Diseases and conditions of pregnancy

Pregnancy-related diseases and conditions

26

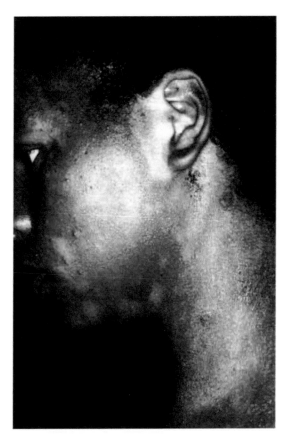

Figure 26.1 Atopic dermatitis, exacerbated during pregnancy. Dermatology Lexicon Project (DLP) preferred term and number: DLP ID: *atopic dermatitis 2100*. Courtesy of Dr T Cestari, Porto Alegre, Brazil

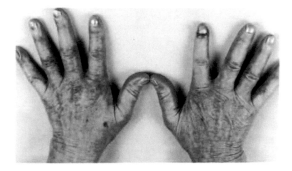

Figure 26.2 Dermatomyositis exacerbated during pregnancy. DLP ID: *dermatomyositis 1796*

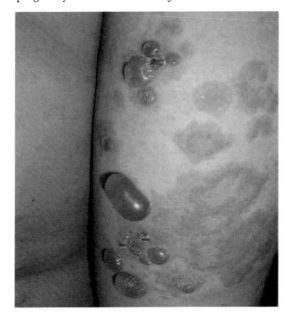

Figure 26.3 Herpes gestationis (pemphigoid gestationis). DLP ID: *herpes gestationis 1762*. Courtesy of Dr S Vassileva, Sofia, Bulgaria

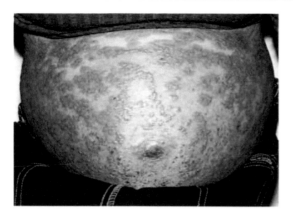

Figure 26.4 Herpes gestationis (pemphigoid gestationis). DLP ID: *herpes gestationis 1762*. Courtesy of Dr M Sollimon, Cairo, Egypt

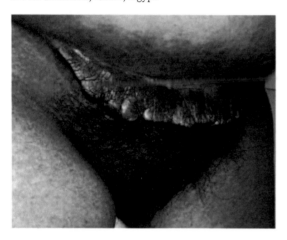

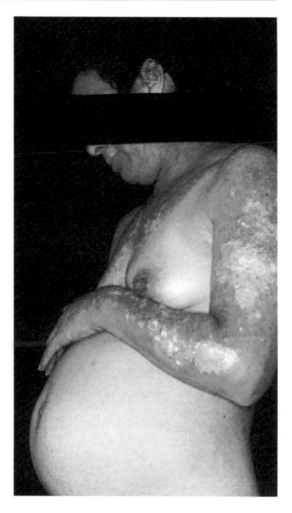

Figure 26.5 Keloids following Cesarian section. DLP ID: *keloid 1264*

Figure 26.6 Lupus erythematosus, systemic, exacerbated during pregnancy. DLP ID: *systemic lupus erythematosus 1808*. Courtesy of Dr T Cestari, Porto Alegre, Brazil

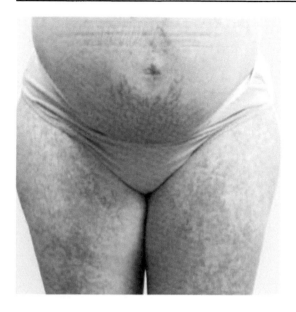

Figure 26.7 Pruritic urticarial papules and plaques of pregnancy (PUPPP). DLP ID: *pruritic urticarial papules and plaques of pregnancy 2183*

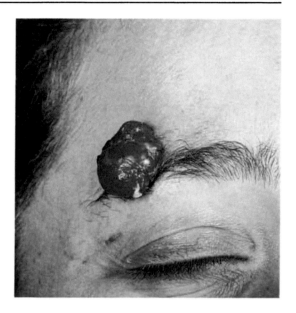

Figure 26.9 Pyogenic granuloma developing during pregnancy. DLP ID: *pyogenic granuloma 2823*

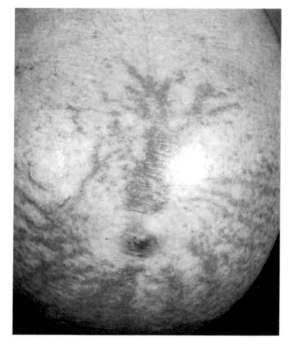

Figure 26.8 Pruritic urticarial papules and plaques of pregnancy (PUPPP). DLP ID: *pruritic urticarial papules and plaques of pregnancy 2183*

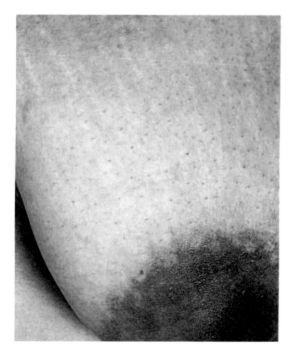

Figure 26.10 Striae distensae. DLP ID: *striae distensae 5223*

Index

Printed and bound by CPI Group (UK) Ltd, Croydon, CR0 4YY

23/10/2024

01777708-0017